GW00729024

THURSDAY'S CHILD

THURSDAY'S CHILD

Stories of survival from a feisty renal warrior

Liz McCue

Waterford Healing Arts Trust

Created through the Waterford Healing Arts Trust programme
at the Renal Dialysis Unit of University Hospital Waterford.

First published in 2017 by
Waterford Healing Arts Trust
WHAT Centre for Arts & Health
University Hospital Waterford,
Dunmore Road,
Waterford

051 842664
what@hse.ie
www.waterfordhealingarts.com

The Waterford Healing Arts Trust acknowledges the financial support
of the Arts Council and Punchestown Kidney Research Fund
in making this book possible.

© Liz McCue 2017

Liz McCue has asserted her moral right to be identified
as the author of this work in accordance with the
Irish Copyright and Related Rights Act 2000.

All rights reserved.
The material in this publication is protected by copyright law. Except as may be
permitted by law, no part of the material may be reproduced (including storage in
a retrieval system) or transmitted in any form or by any means: adapted, rented or
lent without the written permission of the copyright owners. Applications for
permissions should be addressed to the publisher.

Design and typesetting: edit+ www.stuartcoughlan.com
Typeset in Freight

Printed in Ireland by City Print Ltd

Contents

Introduction

Waterford Healing Arts Trust (WHAT) has been running an arts programme in the dialysis unit of University Hospital Waterford since 2007. Artists work in the unit on a weekly basis, engaging patients in art making. The programme, which is funded by the Punchestown Kidney Research Fund, is supported by the staff members on the unit who are keen to provide positive, creative and diversional activities for their patients.

A number of years ago, artist Philip Cullen was introduced to one of the patients, Liz McCue, and together they worked on projects including *Unfolding Time* (2013) and *Tea Room Tales* (2015). Later that year, Liz embarked on a major new journey, supported and accompanied by Philip, to write her autobiography, *Thursday's Child*.

Liz introduced *Thursday's Child* at the fifth Quality Improvement Conference *People Make Change* at University Hospital Waterford (UHW) on 17 May 2017. *Thursday's Child* was officially launched at the WHAT Centre for Arts and Health at UHW on Thursday 8 June 2017.

Claire Meaney
Acting Arts Director
Waterford Healing Arts Trust

Brenda Ronan
Clinical Nurse Manager
Renal Dialysis,
University Hospital Waterford

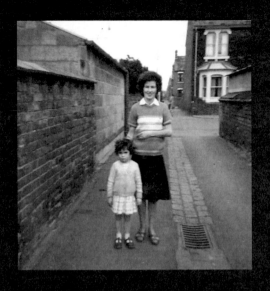

Acknowledgements

Sincere thanks to the wonderful Claire, Maeve, Boyer, Stefanie and all the staff at Waterford Healing Arts Trust for making one of my dreams come true. This book helped me psychologically heal old hurts of childhood and teenage years.

To the Punchestown Kidney Research Fund for the funding to get all the projects up and running for the dialysis patients and for getting my book printed. I have always aspired to be a writer of sorts from an early age. Thanks to the Sisters of Cluny in Chapelizod, Dublin, for their encouragement when I was very young. They believed in me and helped me. My thanks to Brenda and all the staff at the Renal Dialysis Unit at University Hospital Waterford for all your support and care. To Philip Cullen a massive big thanks. Without your hard task mastership, my writer's block and lack of focus would definitely have put me off finishing this healing memoir. You pushed and cajoled me every step of the way. Philip, you will never in a million years know how much this book has helped me come to terms with my demons and to release old pent-up energy from my mind and heart. Thank you also to Jeffrey Gormley for the great editing job.

Thanks to my family, past and present. I love and appreciate you dear ones with all my heart.

To my parents, grandparents, aunts and uncles – RIP.

To the many people who helped me in whatever way they could – thank you all.

From writing this book, I can see that it wasn't my fault that my parents were sometimes dysfunctional due to alcohol. As a child I never felt good enough for my father's love. My mother needed my protection, instead of vice versa. Elizabeth always put everyone first. The only control I had in life was starvation or my other addictions because I was hurting deep inside. I have come to love and respect the inner beautiful soul and the feisty, confident, determined renal warrior that is now the new Lizzybits.

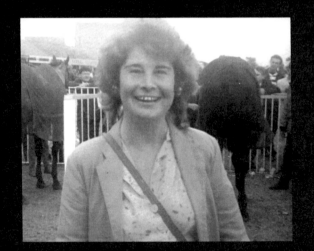

When I was poorly
my Mammy always said
'Elizabeth child, this is your path to walk.
People can walk it with you,
but they cannot walk it for you, pet.
Do your best in life and remember
you have far to go, my sweet child.'

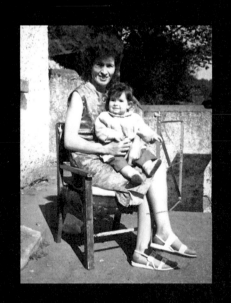

Part One

Rooted in Knockmaroon: My Family Tree

Thursday's child has far to go' my mother often reminded me, and I certainly got a head start! I arrived into this world early. Four weeks early, in fact, on Thursday, 10th March 1960, at three minutes to midnight. I was a beautiful little Piscean, born in the Chinese Year of the Rat to Louise and Albert McCue, but those first weeks weren't easy.

My mother worked for many years at the Jacob's biscuit factory – a reliable job which she loved. She was young and a very dependable worker, a people person and a great mixer with her co-workers. All the staff members called her 'Louie', which she preferred. Most of the staff worked flexi-shift on the different lines, sometimes in the packing department, or on the busy stacking lines, but best of all they loved baking those tasty Jacob's biscuits, because they were able to nibble the odd one or two, when they thought no official eyes were watching. Louie often brought home the broken biscuits that were offloaded at the end of line – 'accidentally on purpose' – so the Smith family always had a biscuit to offer if a visitor called for a cuppa. It was one of the well-known perks of the job.

Louie finished her schooling aged twelve. Always a very clever and creative student, the nuns at Mum's school chose to put her forward to enter a competition for a scholarship. Because of her willingness to not only learn her lessons but help her siblings and others in her class, they thought she would make a great teacher, and, if she kept up her excellent school work, this scholarship could help her achieve a higher diploma, through attaining the honour of attending Mount Sackville School as a day student. That would have been a great achievement – not many children had the brains, nor their parents the money, to acquire a higher education. But young Louie had one, and a chance at the other.

The Reverend Mother arrived up to my mother's class from her private quarters in the big convent. They spoke in private outside the classroom door. It was explained that if Louise's parents allowed her to sit for this big examination, then the clever student had a great chance. Reverend Mother told her to run home and give her parents the wonderful news. A big grin in her mouth, Louie did a few buck leaps as she ran along the road, but when she told her parents 'the wonderful news' she did not get the response she expected. No. 'Louie child', said her father, sitting her down. 'There will be no scholarship place for you girl. Get that notion out of your head, because we need you to bring in a few extra pounds each week'.

The nuns were crestfallen for young Louise. They called to the Smith household and tried to talk reason to Ned and Lizzy, telling them what an honour it would be for their talented and clever daughter and, if she were to win, the honour would go to the nuns who taught her also. They had great belief in Ned's daughter. But once Ned had made up his mind, that was it – 'No' meant 'No. End of story'. Ned hated doing this to his second oldest girl. Louie was always the apple of his eye. Feisty, quick-witted, she took no prisoners in her younger years. She was certainly not happy with this harsh decision from her father, but Ned just didn't want his daughter getting above her station with notions of going to college and leaving home. 'That child's far too big for her boots,' Ned said to his wife, after Louie's cheeky backlash at him.

Louie knew that money was tight in the Smith household; any extra few shillings the youngsters were paid would keep bellies fed and put coal into the small grate in each room, on the rare occasion that they'd be lit – a blue moon or bitter cold, say! Louie knew the next step for her was going over to work with her mother as a live-in childminder for the aristocratic Moyne-Guinness children in the big house on the grounds of the famous Knockmaroon estate.

The Guinnesses were a prominent aristocratic Anglo-Protestant family of bankers, politicians and brewers. The honorable Sir Arthur Guinness was one of the founders of the legendary brewery that made dry stout and porter. He set up in a small workshop on James Street in 1755. A pint of the black stuff, as it's called, was thought to be made from the water of the Liffey, but it's actually from Celbridge spring water, to which is added barley, malt extract and brewer's yeast. The barley is roasted first – this is how Guinness gets its dark colour and taste.

Two Estates

The two Guinness estates were in Castleknock. The main stately mansion, on the Iveagh estate, built in Henry VIII's time, was surrounded by lovely mock-Tudor gate lodges. Across the road was the Moyne estate, where Louie – my Mum! – and her family worked and lived. These two Guinness estates were a big part of village life for Castleknock and Chapelizod, keeping many locals in much needed employment, as well as providing a roof over their heads. My Nana Lizzy worked as a domestic servant, like her mother-in-law Bridget Smith before her. There were always beds that needed changing, dinners to be cooked, or washing to be done. Having her young daughter (my aunt) Biddy working with her was a great help for Lizzy Smith, who could stay in the kitchen where it was warm and rest legs that suffered bad varicose veins. Young Biddy could run like a ferret after a rabbit to do the jobs that needed doing, such as polishing the huge great hall and stairs.

When any 'big noises', as Lizzy called the dignitaries, required someone to light their bedroom fires, or whatever else they wanted doing, a loud bong would sound upstairs. The antique brass gong hung proudly on its impressive stand, complete with the big beater. It was bought in Kenya and shipped home from one of his Lordship's many wild and wonderful expeditions. This was Farmleigh House, an awesome mansion with many staff members, on the massive estate of the Earl of Iveagh, Lord Benjamin and Lady Miranda Guinness. This estate included a huge farm, with dairy cows, horses, pigs and sheep. There was a big lake with a boathouse well stocked with leisure boats for the gentry who wanted to relax on a peaceful afternoon and a picnic hamper which would be freshly made up for their boat trip.

My great-grandparents Matthew and Bridget Smith had moved into a gate lodge in Knockmaroon in the early 1900s. This is their true and sad story, as told to me by mother:

Matthew had a good education and when he finished his schooling was employed on Lord Moyne Guinness's family estate. His was a well-paid and important job: sole charge of the big electric generator, a magnificent device that converted mechanical energy into electrical energy. It was needed to keep the residence well-lit for the Guinnesses. Matthew was a handsome well-turned out young man. He soon fell in with a lovely, jovial lass with long vibrant red hair falling in ringlets down her back and a nice slim waist, though she was curvy too. Bridget's twilight turquoise eyes, with mischievous glints of laughter and fun, gave young Matthew a pep in his step, and it wasn't long before he set out to capture her heart, which in those days meant putting a ring on her finger.

Bridget was a devout Catholic girl, always going to Mass when work permitted. Matthew was born and brought up in Palmerstown by well-respected, wealthy Protestant parents. It did not take the two long to fall in love. This didn't go down well with Matthew's parents. They were very strict, and frowned on the mixed-belief couple getting wed. It was not common for Catholics to marry Protestants, but as the saying goes, 'love knows no boundaries', and some young people were willing to be shamed by excommunication from their parishes. None of Matthew's family turned up on the big day. It's terrible that religion can make people feel sad on the happiest day of their lives.

Matthew had to take his lovely new bride Bridget away from his own neighbourhood, so they moved into one of the lodges at Knockmaroon. The Lodge was situated in a beautiful leafy landscape, surrounded by woods and lush green fields. The rent was included in their salaries. Bridget was employed as a parlour-maid in the big house, and Matthew continued working the big electrical generator. In the evening he would welcome at the gate callers-in visiting the Guinness family on the estate.

Bridget liked her new job. Before, she had worked in the Stewart Institute as a kitchen worker. In this new domestic job in Knockmaroon, you name it, Bridget could turn her hand to it. From early morning until late in the evening, whatever needed to be done in the house, she worked tirelessly, and with pride, doing her many chores or serving for one of the many functions the family held – big banking conferences, yearly harvest festivals, the annual Hunt Ball and of course Christmas extravaganzas. Late at night, Matthew might be called upon to open the estate gate to let the gentry out.

It wasn't long before baby Edward was born in 1911. Named Ned for short, that was my grandfather.

The Poacher

Granda Ned liked school. Being young and agile, he often took over his Dad's duty opening and shutting the gates late into the night. His first job was at the Palmerstown Ink Mills. A true swashbuckler was young Ned Smith, a tall and very straight-backed, athletic lad. With jet black, shoulder-length hair and his rugged distinguished looks, he was very handsome. Ned loved the girls and they all loved Ned. Oh yes, a bit of a boy was this young fella, and he knew it.

Ned loved to go fishing at the Strawberry Beds weir and further along the banks of the River Liffey. He always spent his money wisely, buying fishing tackle to feed his hobby. First a rod, then a big fishing net to catch the salmon or sea trout, a plain spike, and he was always buying floats and bait hooks. He would spend ages digging up worms to tempt the fish nearer the floats. He often caught big conger eels, both brown river and white sea trout, pike and other river fish. But Ned's favourite sport, along with all the other Mill men, was poaching salmon. They would throw the net across the weir when the salmon would be coming upriver to spawn, those same fish having swum all the way across the

Atlantic from the Sargasso Sea off the north-eastern coast of Cuba, all the way back to their nursing grounds in the same hole in the riverbed of the Liffey where they had started off as tiny eggs.

Evading the water fisheries bailiffs at the Liffey weir was the challenge for Ned and his many fishing pals. That gave them their adrenalin buzz. They would meet up afterwards and have a few pints in the Angler's Rest, sharing their many stories and snippets of gossip. They would laugh their hearts out at how they had beaten the 'Billy Bailiffs' yet again.

Eventually Ned met his bride-to-be, Elizabeth O'Neill. After their wedding, Lizzy, as Ned called her, moved from the lush Strawberry Beds to live with Ned and his parents at Knockmaroon Lodge. After a year or so she conceived their first child. In fact, Lizzy was expecting a set of twins, but after the first baby was born, named Bridget in honour of Ned's mother, the doctor told Lizzy there was a complication. They needed to act fast to save both mother and child, so they rushed Lizzy to theatre and performed a Caesarean, a procedure which I believe left my granny mentally scarred for life. Sadly, the baby boy was stillborn, and immediately taken away and buried in an unmarked grave. How sad this was for my dear grandparents, I can only imagine. Lizzy didn't once see the stillborn baby who had grown nine long months in her tummy.

Baby Bridget was very fortunate to have lived, but she grew to be a fine sturdy baby with a good head of reddish hair, like her namesake grandmother. Called Biddy for short, she was joined two years later, in 1932, by baby Louise. Then, at last came the longed for boy. His parents never did get over losing their first son, but Lizzy was over the moon and Ned very proud to have another Edward Smith to carry on the family name. They nicknamed him Neddy. Baby Elizabeth, born in 1940, was called Betty. The names were all shortened in the lodge!

The last sturdy and feisty little baby came in 1943. That Patty could walk before she could crawl was the standing joke in the Smith household, God bless them all. Grandmother Bridget brought up Lizzy's children for her, she being employed fulltime at the big house. Old Bridget was getting on in years and taking a deserved rest from the heavy chores at the big house. Both grandparents were getting old and unwell. By the time Bridget died with a bad heart and a massive stroke, her husband Matthew was deaf and slightly daft. He would ramble on in his well-educated voice about things that happened long ago that never made much sense to the youngsters. He suffered terribly with stomach problems and the grandchildren had to walk the three miles to Chapelizod Village for his stomach antacid tablets. It was a sad time for the Smith family, as the children loved both their grandparents.

Matthew died in terrible pain. Soon after, the nightmares began. The family often complained that the lodge was haunted. No one would stay alone in the house overnight. Each one had a story to tell about mysterious comings and goings in the lodge. There were sightings of shadowed figures and sounds of footsteps walking around upstairs. As far as rattlings in the night goes, my guess is that the mice were doing a flamenco in the food larders!

The Gambler

When Ned Senior was working in the mill in Palmerstown, he couldn't open the gates, so young Neddy Junior (my uncle) took over. He loved his little job, it made him feel important, and often the gentry would tip him with the odd few shillings. Neddy used the money to back a few 'nags' in the bookmaker's office in Castleknock village. He was too young to go in himself, and he couldn't write properly due to dyslexia, so he would get the men to bring out a few betting slips and a pen, and the sports page with the runners and riders on it. The men would put the bet on for him. Neddy picked his horses at random, but he often had a lucky win. Ned Senior also loved backing horses, but his aim was to win money. Like all young lads, Neddy liked to copy his father. It made him feel grown up.

Any few bob Neddy won on the horses was spent first on five Woodbine cigarettes. He would get his friends from the bookies to buy them in the shop. Then he would swagger over the road to the public house. There he would stand, outside, swigging from a small bottle of beer. He always kept one eye on the road, in case his mother, or one or more of his sisters, came along. The girls would be sure to tell his mother, or worse still, his daddy.

Sometimes when Lizzy got hold of him, she would frog-march the young fella home by his earlobe, giving out lingo all the way. 'The disgrace of a young scut like you drinking outside the pub, if you don't mind', she would be saying. Neddy would be mortified with the shame of his mother marching him along like a bold child. Ah, Neddy loved trying to act big and butch in front of the men in the village, but he was a harmless, inoffensive young fella. In fact, everyone loved young Neddy, everyone, that is, except the Christian Brothers in the boy's school.

The Christian Brother teachers were very cruel to young children and Neddy hated them for it. They belted the living daylights out of him, and he often came home battered and bruised, with a bleeding nose, crying in pain, unable to sit down, only for his dad to give him another few skelps for 'good measure'. It was always the way that if the nuns or the Brothers gave any child a beating, it was guaranteed the parents would believe the higher authority before their innocent children.

The nuns and Brothers could be brutally cruel to the poorer children that they thought were slow learners or just plain stupid. Dyslexia wasn't heard of in those years. Neddy and his oldest sister Biddy both had slight learning difficulties and they were always picked on, getting the strap or a few belts on the head from the teachers. Louie hated to see Biddy sore and bruised, so she would help both her sister and young Neddy by doing their homework with them, trying to help them as much as possible. When Louie and Neddy were sent to Castleknock College to get the big milk urn for their mother every night, Louie brought a boy's magazine to read it for her brother under the light bulb on the street. He loved *Dan Dare* and his escapades. He would keep asking, 'Louie go on, read more for me Lou, ah please. Lou, another page before we go'. They often got told off for dilly dallying along the road in the dark.

Biddy needed help with her reading and sums, mostly. There was one nun that particularly disliked Biddy. If she got near her, she would let a swing at her or grab hold of her beautiful long red hair. Louie would tell her mum all this. One day Biddy came home pumping blood from her nose. Lizzy had had enough. She stormed down to see the vengeful nun at the school and let her tongue roll at this old rip of a nun. Bridget was very special to her mother Lizzy, because she knew how lucky Bridget was to be alive.

When he finally left the school in Castleknock, Neddy went to work for Lord Benjamin on his estate, learning his way at the landscape gardening. His Lordship got the Don of the estate to teach Neddy the different flowers, fruits and shrubs. This job was a great start in life for a young lad with dyslexia. Neddy was delighted. No more terrible beatings from the Brothers in Castleknock, or trying to learn lessons he just couldn't understand.

Notions of Grandeur

Louie – my Mum, remember – was taken on as a childminder for Lady Elisabeth Moyne's young children. There were three small infants to mind. One baby was still in the pram, while the other two were a handful to keep up with, but Louie enjoyed minding the children. It was a challenge which kept her on her toes and she loved it. The money, though, was too poor for her liking – Louie had notions above her station, even then.

One day the Guinnesses took her and her sister Biddy to Biddeston House in Andover, a big mansion on the grounds of their estate near Ludgershall Village in Hampshire, England. They lived there in the winter months. Louie liked this new adventure, away from home in Knockmaroon.

Over in Biddeston, the domestic staff got a day off every second Wednesday. Louie relished the afternoon off. Working for the Guinness family gave her ideas of grandeur, so she would spend a while looking at all the new fashions in the window of the local boutique, and then have afternoon tea in the pretty little tearoom on the main street. Louie always treated herself to a cream bun, or a wafer thin sandwich with ham and cucumber, as befitting a 'lady'.

One Wednesday, while out prancing around in her new high heels and Sunday best, with a brand new pair of stockings on her pencil thin legs, she was having a quick glance at her reflection in a shop window pane, when suddenly she tripped and fell on her backside. The young girl was mortified and very upset, as well as having a long ladder in her new stockings. A few people helped her to her feet. Oh the embarrassment of it all! She was on the verge of tears when along came a handsome young lad – dark brown hair, blue twinkly eyes, a lovely deep smile. He was a bit on the brawny side, strong and muscular, with an all-year tan. Louie later learned that this young man worked as a stable-hand on one of the other nearby estates. He had seen Louie fall, and helped her to her feet. After enquiring how she was after her misadventure, he invited her to join him in the tearoom!

The waitress brought a pot of Earl Grey and two delicious cream cakes to the table where they sat pleasantly chatting and getting to know each other. Louie was delighted she had met her first proper fella. He introduced himself as William Eddowes – Bill for short. Now Bill liked his few drinks and wanted to go for one or two with Louie, but she realised that she was too young to go inside a public house. She was worried, too, in case her employers might get word of it. So the first time they went, they slipped into the snug where it was nice and quiet. Surely she wouldn't be spotted, thought Louie, as she tried a small port and lemonade with ice and a slice of cut lemon. It tasted so good as it slipped swiftly down her throat. The second drink, though, she sipped to savour the lovely taste and to feel the warm tingling in her heart from the port. She liked the feeling it gave her, she told me years later.

More's the pity – that taste got her hooked in later life. On her next day off there was no fancy tea and cream slice. It was a double port and lemon! Bill and Louie had some great afternoons filled with laughter and happiness, and she would count the days on the household calendar in the main hall before they could meet up and go to the warm cosy village pub for those few drinks that warmed her up and made her feel light-headed and merry. The young lovebirds would often go for walks in the long meadow for a canoodle out of sight of prying eyes.

The housekeeper Mrs Nevitt was the woman in charge, and she kept a stern eye on her new nursery maid. It was not on for her to be out canoodling, and coming in 'half tore' and smelling of alcohol. A few times she, or even her Ladyship, caught Louie climbing in the scullery window that her sister Biddy had kindly left open for her head-strong sibling. All domestic hands and staff were to be in by nine at night and the doors would be locked at ten on the dot. For neither love nor money would the crotchety housekeeper open the kitchen door. The girls took no notice of the rule – someone would always leave a window ajar, or maybe stay up to let the naughty offenders in. Louie would wait until the kitchen lights went off, then quickly climb in the kitchen window and raid the larder before staggering up the back stairs to the attic where the younger staff members shared one long dormitory room. This room had six beds, three on each side, with a small locker beside each bed and a few wardrobes for their clothes and uniforms. The laughs and craic out of them all were mighty as Louie performed her shenanigans on the floor to amuse the other girls.

After many stern warnings were issued to young Louie Smith, one night her Ladyship happened to come home early from an evening out, due to a bad headache. She walked into her bedroom, and what did she see in front of her only young brazen Louie Smith, in her Ladyship's finest frilly underwear, with a big boa feather wrapped around her neck. After visiting the pub with Bill for port and lemonade, she was now gaily putting on one of her mad floor shows for her sister. She was dancing around merrily, but at least she was wearing her own high heels!

Young Biddy had heard footsteps coming and had tried to warn her sister, but Louie was oblivious to anything and everything, so Biddy scampered to hide behind the big loose curtains, out of sight.

'How dare you come into my room and rifle my drawers,' shouted her Ladyship at Louie. Behind the curtain, Biddy started to laugh, and once she started, she couldn't stop.

The laughter set Lady Elisabeth off: she went really mad at the foolish young ones: 'Come out here immediately, whoever you are!'

Louise and her sister Bridget were left very red-faced. No more child-minding duty for Louise Smith! It was off to Holyhead and home on the rough old cattle boat in disgrace. Ned went mad at his daughter, giving out stink to her, for he knew she was the instigator. Biddy was kept on in the big house at Knockmaroon and later returned to Biddestone House with her other young sister Betty, but for Louie there would be no more Bill Eddowes, no more port and lemonade in the local public house, or canoodling and kissing in the long grass, not for this young madam. The lovebirds never even got to say goodbye properly.

The Jacob's Girl

After applying for a few jobs, Louie got a job looking after two small children out in Greystones, Co Wicklow. It was a live-in job and Louie could go home to visit her parents on her one day off in the week. She saved up and invested in a bicycle for herself and would cycle miles. She loved the job, but after the children started boarding school, she wasn't needed any more, so back home she went to Knockmaroon lodge. She kept trying for different jobs around Dublin until she got the factory job at Jacob's biscuit factory in Bishop Street. This is where the famous Club chocolate biscuit was made after the Second World War, as a commemoration biscuit bar. A nice biscuit it was too, coated in milk chocolate with a creamy centre. Chocolate was a luxury in those early war years, a time of ration books and dire shortages of necessary food. Only a limited amount of anything was allocated to each household every week, and chocolate was a *real* luxury.

The girls Louie worked with were great craic, and they had mighty laughs together. She cycled the five long miles into Bishop Street in the city centre, but in the winter months when the weather was cold, damp, frosty or snowing, Mr Glasgow, or Stephen, as Louie always called her 'chauffeur', would come to her rescue. He lived with his wife Eileen and two children in Chapelizod, so it wasn't too far out of the way for his little micro-car. This three-wheeled bubble vehicle was made by Citroën, and the front of the car lifted to allow the passengers to sit in.

My Father

My dad Albert McCue, or Algy as he was mostly called, worked as head bartender in the local public house in Stoneybatter. He had trained for years at his trade. There was a knack to pulling a good pint of Guinness, pale ale, stout or other beer. They always had to be pulled to perfection, and the head on the Guinness had to be 'just so'. Now a head barman, Albert's job consisted of pulling and selling pints and spirits in the public house.

Bartending is a very sociable job, but can also be very tiring. Dealing with people a bit 'worse for wear' with booze, who could be a bit rowdy or even downright rude, was an art. People skills were part of Algy's training and how better to train than in behind the bar itself? Public houses are lively places, for supping or spilling the odd pint, a sing song and maybe the odd fisty cuffs row after a dispute over trivial things. Algy loved his job. The only drawback was that, much as my father loved pulling a good pint for others, he liked pulling them for himself even more. He always had a few pints stored up to have after closing time, tips he had received from happy punters who had had luck backing horses. They would watch the races on the television in the pub lounge, and when their horse won, their winnings would always burn a hole in their arse pockets. My daddy was always treated to a drink by some of these kind regulars. He knew them all well, being from Stoneybatter himself. His father and mother had lived there many years.

Albert McHugh and his ten brothers and four sisters were born and brought up on Manor Street, close to the quays on the north side of the city. One child, Anna, died very young, may she rest in peace. Fourteen children was a lot to raise! Half the youngsters were McHugh, the rest were McCue. This was due to a befuddled Scottish priest who drank too much of the sacristy wine mixed with Paddy Power! Before one of the children's Christenings, he took the name down wrong. In his native Scotland, McCue was the correct spelling to use, so one of the oldest boys kept his real surname, McHugh, while all the rest of the family shared the new up-beat surname of McCue.

My dad Albert and his brothers went to the Christian Brothers School in the city centre. When the McCue boys finished school, they were sent to work in various jobs and trades around Dublin. They worked to help their mother keep the roof over all their heads as Algy's father had died young from a lung disease. They were all fine hard working boys and girls who loved their ma dearly and were a great help to her. She later lost her eyesight thanks to diabetes. It was tough going blind and her recently widowed, but she managed to scramble around her kitchen and bake bread and make big dinners for her fine family.

Algy loved ballroom dancing and often participated on his odd weekend or week nights off. If he couldn't get a lift or a bus, he cycled as many miles as he needed to reach the parish hall where the dance would be held. He was a fine handsome man and always wore his nice suit and tie, with a starched white collar, and shoes that would be gleaming from the polishing they got daily. Algy's hair was a real foxy red and was receding on top; he wore it to the side that was balding.

When Algy lived in Stoneybatter, he was near to everything. But after he married Louie he moved out to 'the sticks' i.e. the Estate at Knockmaroon, so he would cycle home the main Chesterfield Road in the Phoenix Park, more often than not *half-tore* after 'one for the road' too many. It was a very homely house and he was happy to live with Louie and her family. The house was located on the outskirts of west county Dublin, adorned by a big copper beech tree, which gave the lodge a regal aspect. It kept too much sun from destroying the flowers in the beautiful front garden.

The Stanley range was the heart of the home. It was the all-day cooker and was great for keeping the house warm. The kettle was kept on the boil for the numerous cups of cha offered to whoever came in the door. The oven was used to roast the meat, boil spuds and bake pies, breads or apple tarts for after the tea at night.

The top of the Stanley range was also used for making tasty stews and boiling meat such as ham, chicken or rabbit. We often ate rabbit when I was a youngster, until a horrid disease called myxomatosis became rife in the rabbit community in the 50s and 60s. People refused to eat rabbit after the spread of the *myxo*, which caused blindness, tumours and terrible fatigue.

The Stanley range had to be black-leaded every Sunday morning. This was Ned Senior's weekly job, before he cooked everyone their breakfast, the full Irish, as it's called. He would then toast the bread on a fork at the grid of the range grate.

There were three bedrooms. Louie and Algy had the main bedroom, which Matthew and Bridget had slept in all their married lives, before they moved downstairs, due to ill health and old age. If you remember, readers, these were Louie's grandparents. They died long before Algy came along, may they rest in peace. The bed was a king-size antique brass and metal bed, with screw-top brass knobs on top of the bed frame – a great place to hide money, or so Algy thought. The old mattress was made of coarse horsehair. It was a true antique, comfortable and with plenty of room for the newly-weds. Ned and Lizzy had their back bedroom out of earshot and for their own privacy.

Young Patty and her brother Neddy slept in the middle bedroom. On the good days it was plain Neddy, or 'Nedser', as his Mammy Lizzy always called him when he was 'on the love and honour'. This meant he was on the scrounge for beer money. 'That Nedser fella is on the make again', Nana Lizzy would say. He would be looking in her apron pocket, but she always hid her money down her bosom, out of sight. 'Ah go on, ah please. Sure ye know I will give it back to you'. He would torment his mother for a five bob bit for his opening fee to get into Myo's public house. Once he was in there, he was sure to get a few free pints for gardening work he did, or had lined up to do. 'I only want a few bob. To get a pint, please, ah go on, Ma'. God love Nana, she always gave in.

Neddy was well liked for his gardening work. People knew how good he was at landscaping, especially with him working for Lord Sir Benjamin Guinness. He was always as good as his word and paid his mother Lizzy back promptly every weekend, so that in the week that followed he would be able to go *on the love and honour* again! 'There were no flies on Nedser', Nana would laugh.

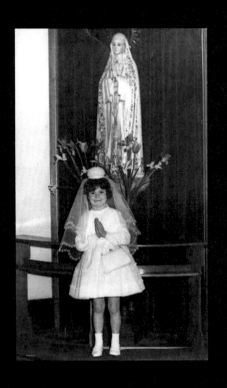

Part Two

Far to go:
My Childhood
in West County Dublin

Knockmaroon Lodge was a busy house with people coming and going to work at all hours. Everyone had a bicycle. This was their only means of transport, that or shank's mare! Having to walk miles meant nothing to the country people and sometimes a passing car driver might stop and kindly offer to give a person a lift. Louie had carried on working well up till near the time of my birth, and really couldn't work anymore. The bicycle came in handy, although it was getting a bit much pedalling in and out daily. Her knight in shining armour, Stephen Glasgow, was now working on the night shift and unable to give her a lift in and out to the factory.

Thursday March 10, 1960, and Louie was getting a lot of pains early in the day. Lizzy was worried about her daughter.

'We will thumb a lift to the doctor in Castleknock, Louie, what do you think?' she asked quietly.

There were still four weeks left before the birth. This was meant to be an April baby, but I made a fool out of everyone. At this stage the pains were wracking my mother's tummy. This was strange for Louie, who so far had had a trouble-free pregnancy. Out they went to thumb a lift to Castleknock Village to see Doctor Nelson. It was just luck that their neighbour Mrs Graham came along and gave them a lift. Louie was in far too much pain to walk the three long miles to the doctor. After he examined Louie, the doctor quickly decided something wasn't quite right with the pregnancy and she needed to get in to Holles Street Maternity Hospital. They managed to get in contact with Patty, Louie's sister, whose fiancé Davey had a car. Louie got a bed in the maternity unit and after seeing a nurse she felt slightly more relaxed. The labour pains were excruciating, coming every so many minutes as I was often told in later years.

Along came the midwife, a big buxom culchie woman, with a pair of hands like shovels. 'Oh God no,' Louie was thinking, 'The hands on yer one are freezing cold, as well as huge.' Biddy was the midwife's name, and the two women didn't hit it off at first. Biddy was rough and not very understanding with her new patient. She had a nurse's watch pinned to her apron, timing each pain as it came along, but after examining the patient her face made a change. 'Wait here, don't move out of that bed please, Mrs McCue'.

Louie was cursing and praying all at the same time. The doctor came and had a look, all business. Next there was great speed, for the baby in Louie's tummy was the wrong way around. Yes, trust me to come out the wrong blooming way, rear end first!

Like with Gran, it was necessary to do a Caesarean; otherwise it could have been fatal for us both. The surgeon had to cut through the wall of my mother's abdomen. After a good while and before getting many stitches in her sore tummy, out popped little Thursday's Child, at exactly three minutes before midnight. I'm told when I came into this world that Biddy, the formidable midwife, got me by my two little legs, turned me upside down and gave me a slap on the cheeks of my bare arse.

'Janey mack', I thought, 'What is this game they are playing at?'

'By God Elizabeth, there wasn't much wrong with your lungs', Mammy told me. 'For a child that was four weeks early, you let a mighty roar out of you, child'. The little baby was a beautiful girl, even if I say so myself, and the first words I heard were Biddy saying to Mammy, 'Your baby girl has long eye lashes and a lovely head of dark wispy hair'.

'Ah she doesn't take after her daddy so,' Louie confided in Biddy, as they sat in the private ward the doctor and sister in charge had decided to give her after the tough procedure.

The midwife was mellowing; in the beginning she had thought my mother Louie was acting up a bit. Before the staff nurses took me away, Biddy put on my little babygro that Mammy's seventeen-year-old sister Patricia had brought in earlier for me to wear.

Davey and Patty found my father after the pubs shut. He had just finished work behind the bar. After Patty explained the full story about my mother going into early labour they gave him a lift to Holles Street to visit Louie and his new tiny baby. They named me Elizabeth after my grandmother on my mother's side of the family.

There I was all snug and cosy in my mother's arms, looking for a drink of milk. Just as I latched on for a nice guzzle from the nipple, in comes another spotty-faced doctor to the room. He thought I looked a bit off colour – I was turning blue! They rushed me to Temple Street Children's Hospital, on the other side of the city. I was put into a little hothouse, what was called an incubator. Double pneumonia was the diagnosis. Sure I never do anything by halves!

Because I was under-developed, it was hard for me to fight this serious infection. Far too small, and not able to cope without antibiotic infusions, I had oxygen tubes put up my nostrils as they tried to keep my temperature level. The incubator was all that was keeping me alive.

The next thing I remember was four sets of eyes looking at me. Two sets each side of my little incubator. Well, I can pretend that I can remember this scene from my baby days.

A few days later, when I was a bit stronger, my parents were let into the special unit to see me up close. I was over the critical stage and out of danger. My parents were told I was a brave and fierce little fighter to have survived the double pneumonia. In another week or so they could bring me home, they were told, providing I kept up the good progress. Daddy was waving at me from one side, and then from the other. I could see my daddy and mother crying. Sure my parents couldn't hear me trying to let them know that I was fighting hard to stay alive. The nurses put me on my back each day and on my side at night. I bet the stench from my nappy was pungent, with all the antibiotics they were pumping into my tiny body. I was fed by a drip until I was able to manage alone. But I was never taken too far from this glasshouse of mine. After four weeks of intensive treatment I got the heave ho – free to go home with my proud parents! They were like peacocks parading me out the door, wrapped in a soft white blanket.

Next, I'm in St Patrick's Catholic Cathedral in the city centre. Oh holy God, the priest tried to drown me. I roared crying in total disgust. Seemingly all new babies needed this procedure, to be drowned by the priest – oops, I mean 'Christened' – after leaving the maternity hospital. My mother told me I looked beautiful in my long white frilly Christening gown and shawl, with my big head of dark wispy hair peeping out. She often spoke about how pretty I looked after leaving the hospital. My father's brother Jack McCue stood for me. This meant he was my new Godfather. Patricia was my Godmother. I always loved my Aunty Patty; she was good to me all through my life, often giving me cuddles and tickles under my baby chin as a small child.

After all the fuss of my Christening, they headed straight to the pub on their way home to 'wet my head'. I was too small to tell them that I had been drowned already, by that priest man!

The Start of My Life in the Pub

There were sandwiches laid on in The Halfway House on the Navan Road. The women went back to the house of Daddy's sister Carmel and Uncle Mick, and left the men to their shenanigans in the bar. Yep, I had far to go. When they eventually got me home to the house in Knockmaroon, there was a dilemma: where in God's name could the baby sleep? I was far too small for the cot or crib. Every place was too big and unsafe for me.

Mammy found the Clark's shoebox she got with the new shoes for the Christening. This was the first place I slept, in my mother's shoebox, still decked out in swaddling bed clothes. This did for the first few nights – it was nothing but the best for tiny little Elizabeth! Next I was put in the drawer of the dressing table for a week, before finally making my way up to the beautiful pink cot they had bought especially for me. It was fit for a princess.

No expense was ever spared, nothing but the very best was got for Louie and Algy's little Thursday's Child. My mother adored me and spent every hour watching over her sickly tot. If I cried, she ran to check that I was okay. Obviously I played merry hell with that arrangement. Maybe all babies do, when they are newly born and full of confidence. Nights at the dances stopped for my parents because Louie would not leave me with anyone, not even her mother Lizzy. This must have been very hard on them both as they loved the parish dances and having a few jars in the pubs. Only for these dances I would never have come along in the first place.

My Childhood Memories

Mr Brendan Behan, the famous, articulate Irish story writer, playwright, poet and stage actor often frequented Myo's in Castleknock. After his busy day walking the boards of the Abbey Theatre, or sitting down at his desk writing his latest short story, he would escape to the village.

I was very young at this time, around three years old. I can still see this distinguished looking man with his long grey mackintosh and a fine head of black, gelled, but dishevelled hair. Brendan always cursed in a fluent tongue. He would always give me a big brown penny from his grey overcoat pocket. I don't remember much about this kind gentleman, but he was a good singer, with everyone applauding him after he sang. They often let out shouts of 'Encore, Brendan, encore man!' He was widely known around the Dublin pubs and in Ireland for great stage performances. He loved his pints of porter and died a young man in 1967 aged 41. What a terrible waste of a gifted man.

Daddy often had a pint with Brendan. They shared a liking of the porter and spoke about pleasantries. When I hear of Brendan Behan, I always think of the big brown penny and a Peggy's leg from Molloy's sweet shop. The pub scene was sad after the quare fella died, RIP Mr Behan.

Over the first year Mammy was always taking me to the local doctor with awful smelly nappies. The urine would scald my rear end. I needed antibiotics every few weeks. I was always a sickly tot. If someone sneezed in my direction then I caught their cold. Over the years I had everything going that could be got, illness-wise. The doctor was run off his feet with me. If we could not get to him, then he came to me. My Mammy was a bag of nerves with me and my long term sicknesses. When I was well, she always brought me out to show off to people they knew. She would be proud as punch pushing my posh blue pram with the relic of St Therese hanging on it. The pub landlord's kind wife Mrs O'Byrne bought the holy relic for me when I first had the double pneumonia. The woman had Masses said for me too, Mammy told me.

When I wasn't sick, life was good. I loved going places in my pushchair. After learning to walk and talk reasonably well, sure, there was no stopping me. I was into everything. 'Curiosity Jane' they could have called their child Elizabeth.

Grandad had great sport with his little grandchild. He was my 'Jamjar' – I couldn't pronounce 'Grandad'. I adored my uncle Neddy, too. Whenever my parents brought me on holidays to Mammy's sisters in England, I would cry every night wanting to go home, I missed them so, doggies, cats, chickens and all. This week or two away always upset me. One time Mammy and Daddy brought me over on the Liverpool cattle boat to visit Aunty Biddy and family. It was a very rough and choppy crossing. Daddy stayed in the bar for the night but he had gotten an overnight bunk for Mam and me. I was on the bottom bunk, and thank God I was, because I fell out of my bunk during the night. The fright I got. We had to double up in my bed.

I loved the parks with swings and slides, and my cousins would mind me and buy me sweets and Tizer – not Sláinte, the Irish red lemonade – and I used to get these ice lollies in the lovely Polish shop that was near to their house. I would be so happy to return home from those holidays. Neddy would be sitting in his chair waiting to see me and of course he would be three sheets to the wind on pints of Guinness or lager. I never cared, as Neddy was nice to me when he got drunk. I'm sure my father felt a bit left out most of the time. He would be pulling a face when I was all over my Uncle Nedser. I was over the moon to see him. I would throw my arms around him and Grandad – provided he was not drinking. I knew to watch out for that. I was a clever little cookie, my Nana said.

She never liked it when all the family got together. They always got very drunk. The way it turned people from mellow to wild and abusive made her unhappy. We would both be on red alert, Nana and I, ready to run for the door and gallop quickly away because as sure as eggs, all hell would erupt. My dear Nana was never a big drinker; a port and lemon or a glass of Shandy was her tipple. One port and lemon and she would sing a song. A great woman was my beautiful Nana Lizzy Smith.

One night after my Uncle Neddy had been out drinking, he came home 'a bit worse for wear'. There was a hawk nesting in the tree in the back garden. Ned Senior owned a double-barrelled shotgun for hunting. It was locked in the wardrobe in the back scullery, out of harm's way. Neddy found Grandad's key. The family were never allowed to touch Grandad's double-barrelled shot gun. Neddy, feeling brave after his skinful of spirits, sneaked the gun out the back door and started shooting at random up into the tree where the hawk was tending her young. Bang! Bang! Bang! Grandad ran out the back, fuming, and a mighty fracas broke out. A few skelps were pulled on my uncle. Grandad had a terrible temper, and drink made him worse. Neddy would have had a lot more bruises only for my Daddy Algy dragged him off. Well it sobered Neddy up. We were thanking God Grandad didn't have too much to drink and certainly no Paddy Power Gold Label!

Neddy didn't dare touch that gun again in a hurry, but another night didn't he come home with a canoe! 'This is for Elizabeth and myself', he said. 'I bought it for the child'. Sure, God bless his heart. How he carried it or who he bought it from, no one ever found out.

Childhood Years – Schooldays

I was up early for my first day at Mount Sackville Girl's School. Mammy had bought Ready Brek breakfast cereal for me. It was a tasty oat cereal that she made in the small pot with milk and a teaspoon of sugar to warm me up, she said, washed down with a cup of tea. I looked well turned-out in my new red jumper and blue skirt, white socks and new school shoes. I had a navy blue gabardine coat to keep me dry when it rained. I felt very important with my school bag and box of sandwiches, my books and pencil case, but as we got to the main school, my nerves finally got the better of me.

The size of me, no bigger than a midget, my mother told me. She brought a packet of Kleenex tissues, just in case one of us might need a cry. I'm sure she was the only one that did, because as soon as we got to the babies class, out came this nice friendly-looking nun with glasses on her nose.

'I'm Sister Aloysius, child,' she explained to me. 'I'm your teacher.'

I wanted to tell my Mammy Louie that the nun had no hair, but I was afraid and just kept quiet. I toddled off inside with the nice nun. Mammy rushed off with the Kleenex hanky up to her eyes. All I wanted was the toilet, as when I got nervous I always needed my wee wees. Beside the main gate of the convent was our public school. Further along the avenue was the private fee-paying school for the boarders and day-school girls. These girls were always driven to and from school by their parents or home-helps – no public school transport for these young ones! There was the public bus for our transport, morning and evening, but I was lucky to live near enough to walk there and back.

Ah God! Truth be told, I never liked travelling on the bus with those other girls as I was a bad mixer due to being very shy. I disliked the other children teasing me or even looking at me. I never knew what to say to them. When they spoke I would clam up. My mouth wouldn't open to utter even a syllable. To get on that bus always made my tummy feel utterly sick. All was grand until it rained very heavily one morning, and I was put on the school bus to make sure I was dry going into class. When the rain was light, Mammy brought her umbrella to keep us dry walking the short distance down to the main gates, where she would kiss me on the rosy cheek and wave goodbye. My two friends Phyllis and Veronica would wait at the main gate, and we would run in to the cloakroom together.

I loved school once I got settled in with these nuns, the Sisters of Saint Joseph of Cluny. I got very attached to them. They were kind and caring to all of the girls, and I learnt a lot from my early years with them. I started off in the infants class, as it was called. Mother Aloysius was our teacher. She was a very motherly nun to us babies and would wipe our noses or plait our hair if it ever came loose from the ribbons. I learned my prayers, how to knit and crochet, how to draw or make pretty pictures, count to twenty and I learned my times tables from two upwards. I even spelled my own name; that was a lot for a little one no more than a midget. Even Mammy was proud of her little Thursday's Child. I loved Mother Aloysius, and she was fond of me, taking me under her wing with an extra class in reading after school when I moved to second class.

For lunch we all brought sandwiches to eat in the playground or the shelters, made in the summer with Nana Lizzy's fondly made strawberry or raspberry jam – whichever fruit she could pick from Grandad's lush, overflowing garden. He grew flowers, fruit and veg throughout the year. Whatever he could get his hands on to plant was grown to perfection out in the back garden. We were blessed, Nana used to say, because we were self-sufficient in those days. On one of the poorer days, lunch would be *uggy*. Yes good old bread and sugar sandwiches, or maybe a bit of dripping. On a really good day, it might be a bit of Dublin cheese and a ripe one from the stems of the tomato plants, if the sun was really shining over our house.

My favourite nun was Sister Brendan, who looked after 3rd and 4th class girls. Sister Brendan could blow hot or cold in the mornings because of her unpredictable temper. Then her stern and grumpy mood might turn jovial and funny in the afternoons. I'm not sure, but I always put it down to the 'message' she got from The Anglers Rest – more of that later.

The morning ritual was 'the Sister Brendan march'. She would stride up and down the rows of desks, enquiring as she went at each girl's desk had we got our homework finished. She always had a cross and stern look on her face. My ear stuck out on the left because of something to do with my time in the incubator at the hospital as a baby – I was put lying on my left hand side and the ear bone grew out of shape. When Sister Brendan got to my desk, her fingers automatically went for my big ear: she got her thumb and index finger ready to tweak it as hard as she could. I pretended it didn't hurt me, but honestly, I felt the pain. Tears would be near to my eyes, but I was damned if I would cry like a baby. I always had my homework done, neat and tidy for her close inspection. On Monday to Thursday evening, Mammy sat down with me for over an hour to help her nearest and dearest with her exercises. I would read my English book, then practice my times tables, geography, history, spelling and catechism. But weekend nights were a definite no-go for her helping me with my learning, due to Mam being on the booze.

Sister Brendan often kept me back to help me learn even more. She knew I loved to read my book, I loved spelling and also I got help with my vocabulary, in other words, an elocution lesson. My mother was always pleased with school reports from old 'Squeezy Ear' Sister Brendan. I was blessed to have her looking out for me, and was happy to be her teacher's pet. I had to collect each girl's copy book for Sister to mark our homework, and I was the obvious one to get her brown paper bag 'message'.

Not many children ever went to pubs, but I'm sure Sister Brendan knew my Daddy frequented the local pubs, and that I knew my way to The Angler's Rest. Any morning that I was sent on this errand to Larry O'Byrne's bar, Sister Brendan would first call me to her desk.

'Elizabeth, I need you to do a message for me child.'

She would give me a neatly folded note to give Mr O'Byrne – the note always had money inside it. I was given strict instructions not to lose this note and to mind the change coming back to school. Money was usually short with the nuns.

I would then set off and run like the wind, or at least as fast as my legs could carry me. That way I could have a sit down at the wooden table and benches outside the pub. There was a parasol umbrella which I could sit under. I sometimes got a packet of cheese and onion crisps and maybe an Aztec bar – a lovely chocolate biscuit bar with peanuts inside, plus, if I was really lucky, a bottle of Coca Cola or Club Orange to wash them down. That was of course if Grandad Ned, or his friend Tommy from Chapelizod, were in the bar for a drink after their early poaching on the Liffey and were feeling generous. They would have one pint before going home to show off their catch, which could be a sea salmon or trout. We'd have it that evening for the tea.

Sometimes I would sit too long and would have to fly back up the road to school. I often pretended that I had got a bad stitch in my side and needed to sit down on the path to have a rest. I'm sure Sister Brendan believed me, or did she just give me the benefit of the doubt? Anyway, she got her much-needed 'message'. What more did she want?

Sister Brendan would always ask me to knock on her classroom door and to wait outside until she came out to me. I was never to bring the 'message' *into* the classroom or to leave it with the secretary. I was to always stand there waiting until she came and took it from me personally. It would be nearly lunchtime. After the bell was rung, the kids would come charging out of the classrooms. Sister Brendan would come out all smiles and thank me for getting her message. The hour-long lunch break in the office would transform her. It was just as if someone had waved a magic wand over her and changed her from a big ogre into a lovely happy smiling nun. Ah, most of the girls loved the Jekyll and Hyde nun.

Summer Holidays at Knockmaroon House

When I was on my summer holidays, my Nana Lizzy often brought me to where she worked to help her do a few little jobs. She worked each morning in Knockmaroon for his Lordship, his wife and family, so some mornings I could go to 'the Big House' and play with the children's old toys. I really enjoyed going places with my dear Nana in general, but the first experience in Knockmaroon House nearly took my breath away: I saw these animal rugs – real animal skins with their awesome heads still attached, including a lion and tiger. Oh my God, it was like somebody had split them and took their innards out. I really expected these animals to growl at me. I would forget that the wild beasts were dead. There was a huge rhino head with its horn still intact up on the wall near the high ceiling. How awful it was to kill these beautiful creatures from God for sport. I always felt sad for these precious wild creatures from lands I may never see.

Each room had lovely woven mats with mohair from Angora goats. There were bright Persian carpets, with traditional woven designs, shipped from Iran or maybe further. They were exotic and very beautiful – it was like going into a fascinating new world: every room could tell a story and each member of the family could, too. In the beautiful luxurious bathrooms there would be a porcelain soap dish for the aromatic *Garden of England* soaps, with hand and body creams to match. The sweet aroma of dried lavender, herbs, spices and other petals would tickle my nostrils. This basket of herbs, called potpourri, my Nana told me, would be put on the window sill. Now I knew my flowers, as Grandad Ned helped me with the exotic names, but I never heard of this potpourri stuff. I did like it.

The big house both amazed and scared me at the same time. The house was haunted too, like many stately homes throughout Ireland. A soldier often marched up and down the winding staircase and sometimes the hooves of a horse and a man's boots could be heard as plain as day. These sounds were heard by many people in the house over the years. The main wine cellar that was underground in this place scared the bejeepers out of me.

One day, Christy, his Lordship's butler, brought me down there to fetch some expensive wine for the big party that was to be held that night in the ballroom. The light was on in the underground cellar and I thought that I would hide on old Christy. The man was stone deaf and obviously he forgot his hearing aids that morning because even though I shouted loudly at him, he thought I was gone! He turned off the light in the cellar. Ah jeepers, it was pitch dark. My heart started bursting out of my chest. Holy God help me. I started roaring crying, and banged on the huge oak door as loudly as I possibly could. I was petrified of the dark and nearly wetting myself in fright, that rats or mice would come out to play with me, locked in the dark, dank cellar. It was very cold down there. I heard the bolt getting pulled back and the light was switched on. It nearly blinded me. Obviously I was in a terrible state. Nana was shouting, 'Elizabeth are you down there child, can you hear me?' They couldn't find me anywhere, inside or outside the big house, and had shouted at Christy to ask if I was with him earlier. When he said 'Yes', the penny dropped with them all – Elizabeth must be still down in the dark wine cellar!

I never went near that dingy wine cellar on my own again, or played silly devils with dear deaf Christy.

Goodbye

I missed doing Sr Brendan's message after moving up to Sister Columbanus' class. It was my second last year with the nuns. I was hoping to excel in my final years and maybe get picked for the free place in the convent as a day boarder. I was doing my best and learning every night with my mother, except for the dreaded weekends when I was taken out on their drinking binges.

Sister Colm, as she liked to be called, explained to us about music lessons. Each pupil could learn to play a musical instrument of their choice: guitar, violin, piano, accordion, bodhrán, or even the banjo. I was very excited to hear this. I wanted to learn the violin. However, a few weeks after moving classes my world came tumbling down – I had to say goodbye to everything and everyone I knew and loved and go to England.

I especially hated leaving my friends Phyllis and Veronica and there was no more talk of learning to play any music. This all left me broken-hearted and feeling gutted, to say the least.

Veronica's mother bought a lovely *Imperial Leather* wash set with soap and talc for Veronica to give me. To this day I cherish the smell of *Imperial Leather*, because after arriving in England, where I often felt very sad, I would take out my talc and smell it. The tears would fall silently; with this reminder of Veronica, my dear friend, I would eventually calm down. I never even got to say a proper goodbye to all the nuns or children in Mount Sackville before we took that jet plane to England.

The Ten-Bob Note

My heart was thumping. It was freezing cold. The frost always made my heart beat faster and took my breath away. It was starting to snow heavily; the east wind had a bitter feel to it. My red nose was nearly raw with the cold from the sharpness of it blowing against my skin. I was near to tears, and fed up waiting like an idiot. I had forgotten to bring any gloves and my chilblains were itching my fingers and toes. As children were not allowed inside any pub after 9pm at night, the barmen made sure that they waited outside. Parents would get told off for having them in the pub. But in the cold late evening, there were never any children except me standing forlornly outside Myo's. This was the usual carry on every Friday and Saturday evening, standing there solitary outside the pub in the village, waiting for the two of them – Mam and my Aunt Sis – to bring me home. I dislike weekends to this day due to these drinking sessions.

Every Friday after school, without fail, I arrived up to the pub to meet Great Aunt Sis and Mam. Aunt Sis would give me a ten-bob note but, by God, this money brought me torture because it helped Mammy to stay out drinking every Friday, Saturday and Sunday. I never realised then that Aunt Sis gave it to me to save embarrassing my Mam by handing it straight to her. She knew I would always give any money I had to my loving mother.

Now that ten-bob note was no good to me, or so I thought. I wanted real money, not a bit of paper in my hand. Little did my innocent childish mind know how much I could have got with all this paper money. I would look at the bit of paper, hand it to Mam, and then wait patiently for her half-empty purse to open. A huge smile would brighten up the crevices of her eyes and lips as she would gladly give me the coins that I preferred so I could go and spend them across the road in Molloy's sweet shop. Sometimes I would get a lovely shilling and a sixpence, and other times I might only get brown pennies. Ah the innocence of youth – sure all I wanted was a Peggy's Leg! That Mr Brendan Behan RIP got me hooked on them when I was small.

The weather never deterred the duo from going to watch the racing on the television in Myo's lounge. It was a good job I had remembered to bring my warm coat as usually I just rushed in home, changed out of my school uniform, and ran up the road to meet them both inside the pub. There they were, sitting in the warmth of the lounge bar, drinking a glass of Guinness and picking out their horses. I don't know why they bothered. They would moan and curse to shame the devil when their nag would come straggling home Paddy last.

Now and then Mam or Aunt Sis would bring me a bottle of Coca Cola and a packet of King Crisps, to keep me quiet in case I would start nagging: 'When are we going home...?' My Mam Louie hated to hear the word home. She would say 'Soon now Elizabeth. Drink your Coke and eat your crisps; sure we won't be too long now'. The horrid smell of her breath from the top shelf spirits was potent. She would have her Bacardi and cokes; Nana Lizzy's sister Julia, or Aunt Sis as everyone called her, would be on the gin and tonic. The gin always played havoc with Sis's moods: when she got very sad, as she did when she sang her few sad songs, the tears would flood the place; but if they won on the horses she would be smiling from ear to ear. God bless her heart, she had lovely soft blue eyes. A very generous woman, was Sis.

So, on this one night, freezing cold, I decided that I wasn't standing for it any longer. I sneaked into the warm foyer and stooped down on my hunkers in case one of the barmen might catch a glimpse of me hiding and put me out in the cold again. I knew all the barmen well. They were very important looking in their white shirts and dickie bows, with dark coloured jumpers and black trousers.

Sometime after half-nine the two women would come staggering out. I could set the pub clock by the two of them. They would be reeling around, trying to hold each other up, and making a hash of it. They were always in the divine horrors. 'It's a case of the blind leading the blind', my Nana Lizzy would say about the drunken duo. It was two steps forward, three steps back, like the ballroom tango dance, the whole way down Castleknock Road. I often had bruises on my own legs from trying to pick them up; one would invariably end up pulling me down also. It was madness for a child my age to be looking after two grown women. It should have been the other way around. I would get them up and we would be on our way, with them both swinging out of my arms. I felt like a rag doll as they pulled me from side to side. Louie said she didn't want me falling on the road and getting myself knocked down. Now that was good coming from her, and she with her feet on the road more than the footpath, three sheets to the wind. I was like their minder in the middle of them, trying to keep my Mam up off the road, and Aunt Sis out of the rat-infested ditch.

It was pitch dark. There were bull frogs croaking in the ditch. What an eerie, deep, weird sound that was. I was terrified in case a big rat would come scurrying after us and attack our ankles. Mam often told me a story about a big black rat attacking her one day as she walked down the road with me in my pram. Why she tried to scare me I don't know. There were miles to walk. I got so tired with both adults hanging out of my sides, but at least I felt brave, facing my fears. I lay down in my warm bed to rest my weary young mind. I knew I had done my best, afraid as I was about bull frogs and king rats and drunk motorists in their cars. I would often wake up shaking and very frightened.

Elizabeth's Liffey Escapade

The River Liffey rises in the Liffey head bog between Kippure and Tonduff, forming many streamlets at the Sally Gap high up in the Wicklow Mountains. It flows 82 or so miles through Wicklow, Kildare and Dublin before entering the Irish Sea at the mouth of Dublin Bay. It proceeds gracefully through Lexlip, Lucan, Strawberry Beds, Glenmaroon, Chapelizod, Islandbridge and in along the quays before entering the Irish Sea.

As a Pisces baby (sign of the fish!) I loved water of any kind. The river, sea, any kind of pool, or even a puddle to splash about in with my wellington boots on, all were heaven to me. Mammy would tell me 'Now Elizabeth, please don't go messing about in them muddy puddles'. Janey mack, did I listen to her advice? Nope. If I was told not to do something, then I would delight in doing it for devilment.

One evening Mam wanted to get the local dressmaker to make me a new school smock. The nuns in Mount Sackville School had changed our uniform code. All children had to wear their new smock over their day clothes to keep them clean, and not have any one person's uniform less fancy than another. We arrived at Kitty Ballasty's house. We all enjoyed a cup of tea and a Jammy Dodger biscuit and then Kitty measured me for my new smock. That done, I spotted Malachy, Kitty's husband, heading off for his allotment over the road. It was right beside the River Liffey. Just before he crossed the road, I caught up with Malachy and asked him could I please help him. He held my hand as we crossed over the road to his big garden. I didn't know what to do with myself. I was afraid of getting bored so I stood chattering away to Mr Ballasty. He spotted a big garden brush and told me to brush the path for him. There was me sweeping backwards, delighted that I was being a great help to the man. I was singing away to myself: 'All kinds of Everything' by Dana, that had won the Eurovision Song Contest the previous year. It was a cold evening and I was putting my back into the brushing, not looking where I was headed. Next minute there was an almighty splash...

I got a mighty fright as I fell backwards into the river! My head went down under the water. I was holding onto that big garden brush for dear life. Down my head bobs again, my mouth and ears full of stinky Liffey water. I was about to go down for the last time. The very last time, I thought. 'Dear God please help me', I prayed in my mind. My eyes were shut tight. I was petrified that I was going to drown. All of a sudden Malachy got hold of the brush, and pulled it in enough to grab my coat collar. Just then Peter, Mr Ballasty's son, grabbed a hold of my arms. He saw it all from their sittingroom window and had run out to inform his father. God bless them both, they came to my rescue. They hauled me out of the river. I was drenched to the skin, like a drowned rat. But this feisty Thursday's Child still had far to go. I lived to fight another day.

My Aunt Patty and her fiancé Davey were next to come to the rescue. Peter Ballasty ran up through the woods to the lodge to inform them they were needed urgently. He caught them just as they were heading out to a dance for their evening date. They brought warm blankets and clean clothes down for me. I was never so happy than to get my little body into their car that night. I was shivering with the shock and cold. I was lucky not to have caught hypothermia in the really cold water of the Liffey. Mam put me to bed after a nice warm wash and a hot chocolate drink to cheer me up. It was great to cuddle up and go to sleep in my warm cosy bed. For a few nights after the Liffey escapade I had terrible nightmares, dreaming that the Liffey had swallowed me right down to the river bed. I prayed often after my escape from drowning.

Legs Eleven – Bingo Belles
Every Sunday, from September through to Mayday, my Mam, her cousin Mae, their Aunt Sis and myself would take the bus into the city centre to Saint Anthony's Hall at Merchant's Quay, for the Sunday afternoon bingo session. No matter what the weather, it was eyes down, and legs eleven for the bingo belles. We had a chanting rhyme for most of the bingo numbers. When the caller called number one, we would all roar 'Kelly's eye'. It was a great laugh! 'One little duck' - number two. 'Cup

of tea' – number three. 'Knock at the door' – four. 'Tom knix' – five. Six : 'pick-up sticks'. Number seven: 'lucky, no legs eleven'. Number thirteen: 'lucky for some'. Eighty-eight was 'two fat ladies'. 'Two little ducks', twenty-two. Every week more lingo was added to the numbers game. We had gas craic. Mam always gave me her old bingo pages, and I would pretend it was my ticket. This made me feel all grown up. At the interval we would have tea and a Jacob's Club biscuit from the little shop, or a packet of Tayto or King Crisps to munch until bingo started again. Some Sundays the local convent sent in a big soup tureen, kept hot on the gas cooker. Vegetable or tomato flavour, this was gorgeous in the cold weather.

People came from far and wide to chance their luck and try to win a few bob. Christmas time at the hall was especially great fun. The prize money was bigger, due to people trying to win an extra bonus for Christmas spending money. The Christian Brothers always put in a big hamper as their prize in the draw. The local Dublin shops, hotels, and big businesses would kindly donate lovely gifts of food, including everything that was needed for the Christmas cupboard – ham, turkey, potatoes, vegetables, stuffing, gravy, wine, spirits, minerals, biscuits, sweets and pickles – you name it, the generously packed hamper would have it tucked in. Even the selection boxes for Christmas morning, and there was always a plastic stocking filled with goodies for the youngsters.

This big draw was held the last Sunday before Christmas Eve. Ah shucks, we never did win any of the lovely hampers, but it was always exciting waiting to see if we might. Mam always bought lots of tickets on the run up to the Christmas hamper draw, as did Aunt Julia and cousin Mae. I would be sent off looking for the ticket sellers to see if I might bring the women better luck. The money that was made on the hamper draw helped to subsidise the St Anthony's soup kitchens, to feed and shelter the homeless community.

The most we ever won was one hundred punts on the 'big flyer'. These were two big one page flyers of bingo numbers. The money was bigger, so these tickets were dearer. One ticket was played before half-time, the other after the main book finished. I remember the night Mam won her bingo stash. One hundred punts was a lot of money!

She brought us over to Luigi's Italian fish and chipper for our high tea, joking to us as we crossed Father Matthew Bridge. It was bitter cold. We all had to put our hands into our pockets to keep them warm. God, I was freezing. We had fish with chips, bread and butter, and a lovely cup of Lyons tea, followed by a Knickerbocker Glory. I was so excited, I thought all my birthdays were after coming at once. When the young dark-haired Italian waitress brought over my Knickerbocker Glory, I couldn't believe that it was just for me. I have only ever had that once in my entire life. Mam brought us in to the hotel after our lovely fish and chip supper for the women to quench their Sunday evening thirst with a few alcoholic beverages. Mae had Irish coffees and Sis had her gin and tonic as per usual. We got a taxi home, right to the front door, from the lovely Ormonde Hotel. No having to play piggy in the middle escorting the two drunken divas home that night!

Usually on Sunday evening it would be straight to the Cosmo House. This was a public house close to St Anthony's bingo hall. Not one of my favourite places to go. We would stop off at a local shop. The old woman there was very nice. She sold lovely crusty bread, and would carve half a pound of freshly cooked ham on the bone. Mae bought the butter, Aunt Sis the mustard. Cosmo House was not nice, because there were blatant drunken women that always destroyed the ladies toilet by urinating on the floor, as well as other undesirable antics. The toilet rolls were non-existent; maybe people stole them and brought them home. Once there was a towel, so shabby and dirty it looked like a floor cloth, with lipstick kiss marks on it. Jeepers, I wouldn't put my hands near the dirty rag, let alone my lips!

I often wondered why Mam and the women ended up going in to that awful pub. Even thinking of it made my tummy heave. Often times I had a kidney infection. Having reflux caused me severe pain in both kidneys. I spent most of my life on antibiotics, and was a puny child due to the kidney disease. This is why I had such a draw to toilets wherever we went. I always needed the toilet for a pee.

There was one woman that came to the Cosmo House every week with her daughter. Philomena was the woman's name, and the young girl was Mary. She was like me in a way, except that whereas she was mouthy and spoiled, I was shy and introverted, being a redneck from out in the sticks. To me, our little village was a one horse hick of a place. One pub, one Protestant church, one Post Office shop, and another shop with a bookies at the back of it. If you blinked, a person could miss it altogether.

Philomena was a lady of the night, as the others called her. I didn't know why she was called this. Old Tom was a regular drinker in the Cosmo pub. He was also one of Philomena's regular tricks. Tom would always buy them a few drinks and a fish and chip supper. This was in part-payment for a bit of what he fancied. Young Mary would be left to sit chatting with me at our table, while Philomena would be gone ages. When she came back she would look like a total wreck – hair dishevelled, lippy all over her gob. Tom would have two big chip suppers wrapped together. If young Mary was very lucky, she was allowed to share a few chips from each wrapper. Often they might have a sausage that they bought her. The smell of the vinegar was delicious in the pungent pub. Tom would have lipstick on his cheek and shirt collar.

Young Mary was a jealous child. If I had the latest new toy from a Moore Street dealer's cart, then she had to have one exactly like it for the following Sunday. She would throw a tantrum and Tom would give over the money just to shut her up. I never realised until I got older that Philomena would put Mary up to this trickery every week. It was more money for an extra few gin and tonics for her. Only in later years did I learn the meaning of 'woman of the night'.

Nana's Mammy 'Big Uggy'

I had Mam's cousin Mae – 'the fairy lady' – wound around my little finger. Yes, Mae really believed in the little people. She had a mystic look: jet black hair, well made up, beautiful rose petal perfume, plenty of hairspray to keep her hair in place, lashings of scarlet lipstick, done to perfection, and nails the same colour as her lipstick. She would spend ages telling me about the fairies, and I was fascinated hearing about them. Her dear husband Willie was petrified to go out in the garden late at night. I think he really believed his wife's weird and wonderful tales. All the family thought Mae was batty as a fruit cake, but I loved our chats. Mae was special to me. Her mother, Molly, was my Nana Lizzy's sister. She lived in Avoca, County Wicklow, near the Meetings of the Water pub, with her husband and their children. This is where Mae was born. Later, she came to live in Dublin with her grandmother Mrs O'Neill – you remember Big Uggy don't you! Don't ask me why she was called Big Uggy – maybe she liked making those bread, butter and sugar sandwiches. Uggy always wore a long black dress, white apron and white bonnet. She loved snuff and always carried a small tin in the front of her apron pocket. She would take a few pinches and sniff it up her nostrils. It was cheaper than buying ten Woodbine cigarettes! The front of Uggy's apron would be covered in the black powder.

On Sundays in the summer season, Uggy and the family sold punnets of strawberries to the day trippers from their front garden. They would sit by the gate and sell to the sightseers that arrived out from the city centre. Some came on ferryboats from the Dublin quays, on their own fishing boats, or by pony and trap. Then there were the walkers, who often walked over five miles for the punnets full to the brim with juicy red, sweet strawberries, hand-picked fresh for them to bring home for their teatime treat. The sloping hills on the banks of the river behind the main houses on the Lower road were covered in strawberry plants. This is how the famous Strawberry Beds got its name. The ferrymen would transport tonnes of strawberries to the Dublin markets, or further afield.

There was always great sport had on the Lower Road. There were two pubs: The Strawberry Hall and, further down near the weirs, the Wren's Nest. In the summertime in later years the HB man would arrive out to sell ice-cream cones and wafer ices. It was a treat for the sightseers sitting on the river bank watching the river cascade over the tumbling weirs, eating their delicious strawberries dipped in creamy HB ice-cream. Sunday evenings, some of the Dubliners folk group would arrive out to the Wren's Nest for a jam session. The pub would be crammed to the rafters with day-trippers as well as the usual regulars. This pub had a small bar and a middle-sized back room, lit with gas lamps. They had no electric lights or even a phone, like it was lost in a time warp. I liked it because I was allowed to play with the four children out on their garden swing, while me Ma and Sis got hammered, singing their lungs out for all they were worth. This embarrassed me big time – I hated to be shown up in the pubs.

Luke Kelly, Ronnie Drew, Barney McKenna and Ciarán Burke, and a few of the boys from the city, would be blasting out on their instruments. They all had their party pieces: Luke Kelly would be singing a few of his beautiful songs for us, like Whiskey in the Jar, The Black Velvet Band, or the beautiful Raglan Road, written by the famous Patrick Kavanagh; Barney McKenna would be on his banjo, and Ronnie was in a class of his own on guitar. Then there was Ciarán. He was a singer and played the tin whistle, or often his harmonica that was always carried in his pocket. The Dublin Balladeers only came out now and again, the odd Sunday afternoon for a spin. O'Donoghue's was their main haunting ground. That's where they all met to play their music before becoming famous.

As I told you already, Aunt Sis was from Avoca. Many years ago, Julia, as she was then known, married a County Dublin man named Frank, a stocky army man. Their son proudly joined the army – like father, like son – but this courageous young lad was fatally shot in battle at 23 years of age, RIP. This destroyed his mother Julia, and her husband Frank, and helped break up their marriage. He became harder to live with. They had another son who no longer lived at home, so Sis left her own home. She got a job caring for an amateur actress that lived on the Strawberrybeds Lower Road. They got on well, and when this actress eventually died, Julia was left a lot of trinkets and other keepsakes. She then moved in with a friend of hers, as a carer, also on the Lower Road.

Great Aunt Sis lived for the weekend, to get the few gin and tonics to help block out the mental pain and ease her broken heart. I was far too young to understand this dear woman's pain.

When I was outside the pub, every time a 39a bus would come out from town, I would quickly dodge behind the pub in case my Daddy, or someone we knew, saw me. All hell would break loose for having me standing outside a public house in the awful weather. I would be hopping or jumping to try and keep myself warm and praying constantly that we would arrive home long before my father did.

This was because I remembered one late Friday night when Daddy was already home before us. He was eating the steak Nana Lizzy had fried for him. The minute we walked in the front door, my father lost his temper. He went ballistic at my poor Mam. The two of them were shouting and giving out lingo to each other. Nana grabbed Towser our dog and me by the hand, and brought us out to the wood, pretending to be walking Towser. We went in ages later, when all the noise had quietened down. Mam made us all a cup of tea as she was sobering up after the big quarrel. We all went to bed. Then Dad came up later after reading his evening paper, carrying his piss bucket, fags, matches and his hipflask full of whiskey or brandy. I was pretending to be fast asleep. Next thing I hear is grunting, moaning and groaning. My parents' bed was creaking, and Mam was whispering 'Aw no stop Albert, the child will hear us'. 'Ah feck her', I heard him reply. I was thinking and praying in my own mind, 'Ah Jesus, no. Please don't let Daddy hurt my Mam.' I really thought they were fighting. I was too afraid to open my mouth in case I made things ten times worse for my dear Mam. Oh God I hated those weekends and the dreaded drink. I always told myself I was never going to drink or smoke.

Elizabeth's Saturday Treat

Most Saturdays, when I got up, the first thing I would do was go to Mammy and Daddy's wardrobe in the kitchen. There would be my big bottle of Sláinte red lemonade with my packet of King Crisps, cheese and onion flavour, and my bar of Cadbury's chocolate. This was my 'pocket money' from my father every week. I loved getting this treat every Saturday morning without fail. Thank you Daddy, even if it was never said enough to you when it was needed.

The Brazen Head Inn

One Sunday evening after the bingo, we found this really old historical pub located near the quays on Bridge Street Lower. The timeworn walls of this olde world pub must have had some interesting tales to tell. The Brazen Head goes back to 1198. I was around nine years of age, sharp as a button and clever with it. There were Sissy and me, heading home earlier than expected. No Mae Byrne tonight. Mae was unwell with an upset tummy. I always missed my fairy friend and her exciting tales. This pub had no proper electric lighting inside; instead they had oil-lit Tilley lamps. When we sat down at our table, the hair stood up on my neck. I was feeling uneasy about these eerie surroundings. I knew well the women weren't drunk, because they were short of cash. They had only drunk one drink in the Cosmo House. That's why we had to go home early – as Mam always said, 'no mon, no fun'. They had come in for a last bottle of Guinness on the way home. I needed the toilet; luckily they had one, even if it was on the third floor. The bartender showed us the stairs and told us to be careful to mind the creaky steps. He gave us a candle. Up the bockety stairs we climbed. Mam went first, then me, and Sis behind, in case I fell in the dark. Through a half-opened door we heard a rocking chair, rocking fast back and forth on the old creaky wooden floorboards. We could all see a man sitting on the chair. He started whistling an old rebel song, The Croppy Boy. After knocking and getting no answer, Mam pushed open the door. In the dim glow from the candle we saw there was definitely nobody in that room. It was empty. The fusty room smelled very damp – unused for a long time.

We carried on up to the toilet. We were all shook up, and the rocking chair was still rocking, backwards and forwards. Yet no one was in that room. When we got back from the toilet, the door was locked. We carried on down the stairs as fast as it was safe to. Mam asked the landlord who the man was in that room on the second floor. He told us that room was never used for many a long year. The door was always kept locked. Yet we could tell him what was in that fusty old room. He told us we weren't the first to say this about that room, that a lot of noises were heard coming from it, day and night. How true this all was we didn't know, nor did we care to ponder too long on the subject. We finished our drinks and left, never to return.

The TB Hospital

It was at that time that my Grandad and my Daddy both had to go into the TB hospital. Tuberculosis was rife in Ireland in the 50s, 60s and 70s. No children were allowed to go up to the tuberculosis ward to visit their parents or other relatives. I was always made stay in the house at the main gate of the James Connolly Memorial Hospital in Blanchardstown. I really disliked staying in the gateman's hut. He would be bringing up horrible phlegm from his throat, and spitting it out of his big gob, the dirty old geezer.

There were loads of rough-looking snotty nosed kids waiting in the guard hut for their mothers. Mam said: 'Keep well away from them Dublin ones, Elizabeth. They might have them nits in their hair'. The clothes were a bit scruffy and faces a bit dirty. One girl had make-up on. I tried not to laugh at her, but she looked like a blooming clown. The gobby mouth from the city addressed me. 'What ya looking at youse?' she said to me, real cheekily. 'I don't know,' I replied, 'There's no label, it must have fell off yeah.' Then I stuck out me tongue and crossed me two eyes at yer one, just for good measure. Well she flew at me and gave me a mighty box in the mouth. She caught my nose too with the wallop. Blood poured down me. My tears fell in buckets. 'I want my Mammy', I roared at the top of my voice. Yer one was trying to get another bash at me for good measure. The guard on duty didn't know what to do with us. He was cursing and swearing like a trooper, calling us two bloody bitches, and God knows what else under his tongue.

Next minute our two mammies came running hell for leather down the avenue. My Mam had a very cross face on her, as did the other child's mother. She had vengeance on her mind, and venom on her tongue. By rights, my own mother was a quiet demure woman. Only the booze, or someone hurting her precious child Elizabeth, brought the lioness out in my Louie. The other woman was the size of a tank, with a gob even bigger. Bertha was her name. 'What's going on here youse two?', she asked the gateman and her daughter. The spits were coming out of her gob all over us. 'Beryl, what's wrong?' She started to raise her tone to a roar in her high-pitched Liberties brogue. Well my mother was having none of these shenanigans. My clothes were saturated in blood, even the new jumper from the St Vinny de Paul's. When she saw the state of me, she told Beryl the Dublin perils to get back to the city centre if they knew what was good for them, else she and her little yoke would be put into the Accident and Emergency very fast!

Yer one and her offspring weren't long heading for the 39A bus. Mam was mortified, and there were no more visits to the James Connolly Memorial Hospital. I was left with my dear Aunt Patty, instead, which I loved. And thanks be to God for small mercies, because nine long months Daddy and Grandad were in the Sanatorium hospital, both very poorly and nearly dying.

The Broken Tooth

My Mam, Nana, Neddy and Patty worked hard to keep the house running. Yes, pawn shops, St Vincent de Paul, you name it, we were thankful for the charity to help keep food in our bellies and a fire in the grate. The odd Wednesday afternoon, a few of the patients from the Blanchardstown sanatorium often sneaked out to the local pub, unbeknown to the nurses. Seemingly 'Spit' Muldoon, the crafty old gatekeeper, kept his head averted. When the men came back, they took him the odd Guinness or a bottle of Smithwicks pale ale, which he was partial to on the night shift, hidden in a brown paper bag. 'To whisht him up, and wet his whistle', as the men often said.

One day, we were in the pub waiting on my Daddy Albert and Grandad Ned to make their escape from the hospital – Nana Lizzy, my mother Louie and me. I got up on the long pub seat to look out the window to see if they were coming. I got over-excited, and started jumping up and down, squealing 'Nana here they are'. As the door opened and in they both walked, down I fell in a heap and bumped my poor head. Oh dear, out pops my front tooth! Aw goodness, I'm going to look gummy. Well, the roars out of me. I was like a wailing banshee.

Mam took me to the toilet and cleaned my face, and then to the nice chemist woman next door to get some ointment for the cut on my head. I was holding a bit of tissue to my top gum, and Mam told me my fairy godmother would come that night. That soon shut me up, thinking of my nice shiney sixpence that would be under my pillow when I woke up in the morning, and I wondered if I could make another tooth loose for these fairies.

In the chemist the nice woman gave me an orange and lemon coloured lollipop.

'What happened to you Elizabeth?' she asked me kindly.

Mam got all my antibiotics in this chemist every few weeks or so for my kidney infections, so the woman knew us very well. I knew not to open my mouth and tell this woman it was in the pub next door that I fell. I knew by the stern look on my mother's face. I told her I fell and banged my head on the pavement when we got off the 39 bus from Castleknock. She asked if we were going up to see the men in the Sanatorium. I had my story well prepared in case the hospital staff found out some male patients were having a few sneaky pints in the pub near the hospital gate hut. They and Spit Muldoon would be in serious trouble. I was given a few extra sucky glucose sweets because I fell and hurt myself.

'She's very nice, that woman in the chemist', I said to Mam as we walked back in to the next door pub. I sat down nice and quiet, as my Daddy was there, and I daren't make noise or I might get a sharp slap on the leg. Daddy didn't like me to be a 'boisterous child', as he put it. 'Don't be bold, Elizabeth,' he would say. He was never one for too much praise! As they sipped their pints and watched the horses running on the telly, Grandad would order: 'Jimmy, send over a whiskey chaser to follow this pint please.' I'm sure Grandad and Daddy were nearly half-flutered going back to the Sanatorium in the taxi. They would get out at the main gate and slowly stagger back up the avenue to the entrance to the hospital.

Dublin in the Poor Times

'Thank God for the Credit Union,' I often heard my Mam saying to Nana as we walked down to Chapelizod on a Thursday evening to pay the weekly lodgement. This office would be really full at certain times of the year: start of school term, Christmas, Easter, First Holy Communions, Confirmations, engagements, anniversaries, weddings. These good old Credit Unions were a godsend to all mothers, daddies or other family members in need of a few punts.

There were also the pawn shops. I remember being brought into the one in Mary Street, Dublin. The grown-ups would bring in their good clothes, shoes, jewellery, fine bone china and any fancy stuff worth a few punts to pawn with the money-lender. The parents brought the stuff in on a Monday, and they could get it back out on a Friday when their men were paid. In the poor times, some folk did not have many good clothes: one suit, one overcoat, a good pair of shoes, leather if they were lucky and, for the men a cap, or trilby hat for getting dressed up for Mass on a Sunday morning. From week to week, the mammies often pawned their wedding and engagement rings, their own nice coat, dress, high-heeled shoes or boots, or even their savings stamps or money book, to put food on their tables, or a pint in their old man's porter belly, depending on the lay of the land. These offices were packed most days, especially Mondays.

The Saint Vincent De Paul, or Vinny-de-Pauls, was another organisation that helped the poor and homeless people around the city. This was often a great help for mammies that couldn't afford to feed their babies, or other children in the household. The old people often got a free bag of coal or a food parcel at Christmas or in times of need, or maybe a pair of second-hand shoes or boots to keep their feet dry and warm in winter. They collected old clothes from the wealthier and gave them to the poorer homes. Only for people like these in Dublin, it would have been even poorer in those times.

Wherever a person could get a few punts, they would. They were desperate times. One afternoon I was told to keep my mouth closed and just listen, as we went into the Vinny de Paul's office on the Navan Road. It was around the time Daddy and Grandad were in the Sanatorium. It was coming up to Christmas time. The next day this same man came to our house with a big box of some sort and suddenly I had new jumpers, one of them a lovely tomato red. Plus I had an extra Christmas present. I cannot remember for sure, but I think it was a Sindy doll. I was delighted with my parcel, but I was not allowed to tell my friends about our jaunt to the Navan Road, as my school friend Veronica lived near there, and her Mam would know we were poor and in need of help. It wasn't our fault that dear Grandad and my Daddy had lung disease and nearly died from it.

Memory Lane – The Mill

Grandad was never the same again after his tuberculosis; both his lungs were bunched, as he said. There was hardly any lung function left. The noise he made trying to breathe really scared me – so raspy, like he would never take another breath again. The wheezing in his chest was awful. He needed medication to keep the lungs open – a big powder supplement made with water three times daily. He never went back to work in the mill in Palmerstown, where he had worked all those years. He had loved the craic with the men, watching the banks of the River Liffey for the salmon fry going up the river to where they were born.

Grandad's Lunches

In the times when he was working there, I brought Grandad his lunch down to him at the bridge that crossed the River Liffey between Chapelizod and Palmerstown. Grandad would cross this river every day, working in the Palmerstown Mill. When lunchtime came around, he walked back across this bridge and waited for someone to arrive with his lunch. When I had my school holidays, I did it every day without fail. We would meet up at the bridge seat. I would bring him his cheese, tomato and onion sandwiches, freshly made, and a flask of hot sweet tea. Every day I would eat one small cut sambo. Towser and me would share this between us. I love sambos with the tomato gone squashy, and loads of pepper to make me sneeze. Nana Lizzy thought by putting pepper on Grandad's sandwich I wouldn't eat any of his nice lunch, but how wrong Nana was, ha ha. Yummy yum yum.

Many the Odd Punch

There was a big weir between the two banks of the River Liffey, at Palmerstown Mill on the south bank and Lower Strawberry Beds Road, near Chapelizod, on the north. The bailiffs were cut-throat, watching and waiting in case the mill men netted the river to get a mighty catch of salmon or white trout before the fish managed to get past this weir. The men would sell their catch or bring them home to eat. The mill men would be out with waders and flash lamps on a good high tide. The bailiffs would wait in hidey-holes to pounce on them. All hell would then often escalate on the banks of the Liffey weir. Many the odd punch was thrown from mill man to bailiff. Bloody noses, cuts and gashes and the odd bruised black eyes, and maybe a few broken ribs were not unheard of on the River Liffey. My dear Grandad missed all these shenanigans after he left the mill. He was now disabled, as was my own Daddy, Algy.

The Evening Paper

A friend of our family, Kathleen, or Mrs Ballasty, lived with her husband Malachy down at the bottom of the wood, just a stone's throw from the bridge on the Strawberry Beds Lower Road side of the Liffey. There was a big fruit field at the side of the lodge. I used to nip down to Kitty's every day after school for Grandad's *Evening Herald* paper. They kept it for us to read. Malachy would bring it home to their own house. He came home for a hot meal every lunch hour. Kitty would have it all dished up for him, ready to eat. He would sit back and read to his heart's content and smoke his pipe and the smell of tobacco was very pleasant to me whenever I smelt it in their house. The smell would linger in Kitty's front room. Malachy would have a good old read before going back to work in the Guinness estates. He was a foreman on the farm.

Towser the dog would wait patiently, sitting by the front door at home until 3pm every school day. I would run in, change my uniform, put my clothes and my coat on and we were gone like a shot down the steps. Towser would carry his lead handle in his jaws. We would run so fast I would get a mighty stitch in my side and would sit on the step to rest. Mrs Ballasty would be waiting at the door for us. I loved Kitty, though to me she was always Mrs Ballasty out of respect. She would have Miwadi squash for me to drink and a few biscuits for me to munch on, or a bowl of thick broth if it was very cold out.

One day when I was down the woods with Towser, along came this young fella, a shady-looking character. The woods were very secluded, and I got a bit of a fright: as usual there was no-one around our wood. I had the dog tied up on the fence where I was playing, happily, jumping the rope. I brought my skipping rope in my pocket most days. I would set a task, and try to jump higher every evening. Well, I'm not joking, the dog nearly choked himself, leaping and jumping, to get after this gurrier. I had often seen the fella before in Chapelizod Village, which was a few miles away from the house. He was a good distance away from home, whatever he was scouting around after. There used to be a lot of quare fellas, sniffing melted down firelighters and taking 'coke', which I thought was Coca Cola, but I learned later that meant they were smoking dope and sniffing substances. So I was right to run like hell down to tell Kathleen Ballasty to watch out, and keep her doors locked. She said that she did spot him out her window, legging it out the gates.

Kitty walked me half-way up the steps and I started running after she left. I nearly passed by Towser with the speed of me, going hell for leather. When I got home I was as white as a sheet; Mam was worried because I couldn't speak due to a bad stitch in my side from running so blooming fast. They were all mad to hear about my escapade. Phew, what a day. To make matters worse, I had forgotten Grandad's *Evening Herald*. He was raging. He walked down himself later in the evening for it, plus he wanted to find out from Malachy if he knew anything about this prowler.

Twinkle Twinkle Little Star – What I loved about my childhood days
When my Nana and I would go out in the garden to play hide and seek from Grandad late in the night, after he came in flutered from the pub, Nana would point up to the stars in the sky. She would always look at the brightest star, the North Star. 'Look Elizabeth, that's my little baby', Nana would say every time the star would blink. When a cloud went by, it seemed like the star was winking at us both, like it was saying 'hello' to us. Even to this day I gaze up to the sky on a bright moonlit night, waiting for Nana Lizzy and her baby boy of long ago to say 'Hi down there, Elizabeth', and give me the odd twinkle, because Nana knew I was like an elephant, never forgetting my loved ones in heaven.

Halloween
This was the memorial of All Souls, people who had died and gone to heaven. The graves would always be well tended and adorned with beautiful floral tributes for dear loved ones already in heaven, RIP.

Youngsters would go from door to door of the houses all dressed up in scary garish Halloween outfits, with false faces and a black sack so people didn't know who they were. Sometimes the children would sing a song or recite a poem, then say 'Trick or Treat'. Mostly they would get sweets, apples, nuts or a few pence in their little bags, which they brought with them to store their goodies. Hector Grey's curiosity shop in Moore Street did well at Halloween. He sold lots of disguises, bags of lollipops and sweets. You name it, Hector would have it for sale. No matter what the occasion, Hector was the man to bring happy days to each child that crossed the threshold of his shop.

For the first two weeks in November, Masses were offered for the deceased members or friends of the family. So, although it was a happy occasion for the children, it was also a remembrance of the dead too.

The Missions

Masses would be held twice daily during the Missions and missionary priests would arrive home from far-flung destinations and tell us the stories about starving children needing our help, and how we could help them by joining the missionaries abroad. I wanted to go out to the Missions when I left school. It appealed to me greatly. We had a local priest who travelled out to the Andes Mountains to look after the Peruvian people and try to bring them peace by joining the Catholic Church. The priests did great work in these countries. Their stories fascinated me. Even today I would have dreams of helping others in far away countries.

Saturday Night Shenanigans

Each Saturday night, dear Nana had a joint of succulent beef in the oven to roast. The aroma of it when Mam and I would get home from the pub! She would be half-flutered and trying to fry my Daddy's dinner. Nana would tell her to go and sit down and rest her legs, and then she would prepare the food for my Daddy Algy. Nana would want us in bed early in case trouble would start between Louie and Daddy.

It was like a time bomb on the weekend for Nana Lizzy. The minute any confrontation took place, my Nana took me by the hand. We would collect our coats in the scullery, put them on and swiftly shoot out the back door. If it was late at night, we headed out to the woods, which were at the back of the house. If it was early in the evening, it would be Chapelizod Village shop, on the pretence of needing butter or bread. Anything to get away from the shenanigans that were going on in the house.

Now most of these blow-ups were over nothing really – too much drink on a Friday or Saturday night in the Angler's Rest. Larry Byrne, the pub owner, would bring Grandad home at about eleven at night, before the pubs closed. It got rowdy at times when the pub doors were shutting, with the odd punch or bottle flying, and Ned was far too old for this kind of trouble. Larry would drive Ned home himself, or else get one of the old drinking friends that Grandad was singing with all evening.

Now Patrick Kavanagh, the famous novelist and poet, got on well with my Grandad Ned. Patrick and his wife bought a house near the Angler's Rest, on the Strawberrybeds Lower Road. He wrote the book 'Tarry Flynn', based on his own life as a young farmer in 1930s Monaghan, and his quest for big fields, young women and the meaning of life. He also wrote the poem 'Raglan Road', which later became a well known song by the one and only Sheriff Street, Dublin man himself, Luke Kelly.

Ned and Patrick had many deep-rooted chats on the meaning of life in the Angler's Rest on a Friday night. The whiskey loosened their tongues, and the pints wet their whistles.

Trouble was the damn Paddy Powers or Bushmills whiskey would torment old Ned Senior. He would get home snarling, and be very abusive towards his family in the lodge. When that happened, I was called up out of bed in my pyjamas to try to pacify him. It would work for a while – Ned would sing and I would play the lids, pretending to be his band. He was a great singer. He loved the tenors John McCormack and Mario Lanza. You name it, he could sing their songs. He always brought home a naggin of Paddy Powers Irish whiskey, to help him sing, he would tell us. As time passed he would get more agitated, forgetting I was in the kitchen with them. This was Nana's cue to get me out of the kitchen before the lids were sent flying on to the floor.

We would be outside for ages. It was often frosty and once there was even snow on the ground, both of us freezing cold. Sometimes he would come out to the back garden to see where Nana was. We were pretending to hide. Nana told me 'Be very quiet now, don't let your Grandad hear us.' 'Why?' I was about to say. Next minute Nana put her hand very gently on my mouth. 'Shhh, Elizabeth'. After a while all went quiet. That meant we could go in for a hot cup of tea. I never understood what it was all about. Only drink stuck in my mind.

I was afraid when people drank too much around me. I felt like a greyhound ready to spring out of the trap after the hare, to get away from any confrontation that ever popped up. Even in later years I have found it hard to cope in volatile situations. It makes me angry. Even a television show is hard for me to watch if there's any controversy in the programme. My heart starts pounding and I reach for the remote control or switch off button pronto.

Belfast

The big CIE coach turned up early at my school. This bus was to take the children on our excursion day trip to County Antrim in Northern Ireland, to feast our eyes on the sights of the beautiful Mourne Mountains, the rugged Antrim coastline, Carrigfergus and Larne, and to see the majestic 40,000-odd interlocking hexagonal basalt columns at the Giant's Causeway.

We all crowded on to the bus, Veronica and myself at the back, with our little bags of sandwiches and a small carton of Miwadi orange to drink. Mam thought I would be delighted going off for the day trip on the coach. Thank goodness Veronica was coming to keep me company. The sound of Sister Columbanus saying the morning prayers as we started on our road trip gave me comfort. The coach was full. There was to be no messing about on the bus. We were under strict instructions, or our parents would be informed about our boldness. I brought a book with me to read, which helped pass the time. It was Laura Ingalls' 'Little House on the Prairie'. I loved these adventure books. On the way up to the coastline, we stopped to learn about the Mountains of Mourne and Slieve Donard, the highest peak. We got up to the border before crossing over the bridge at Lough Foyle.

The day was very wet. There was no let up in the damp weather north or south of the border. There were British soldiers guarding the border. They had guns on their shoulders and looked very scary to us children, which was what they were supposed to do. They searched our bus and let us go. I didn't know why until later. This took the good out of the day. I got a knot in my tummy. Holy God, my tummy was doing somersaults and my adrenalin levels were kicking in. As long as I was at home in my safe cocoon, with my family, surrounded by my pet animals, or at school with all the other girls and my friends,

I felt safe and secure. I disliked change of any sort because it put my tummy out of place, especially hearing on the radio about the troubles up the North.

Off to the north coast. We got out to walk on these big columns of rock formations, left like this after a volcanic eruption many thousands of years ago on our craggy island of Ireland. They were outstanding in their ruggedness.

We went to the funfair at Carrigfergus. We could go on one ride. Veronica and I went on a swinging boat, her on one side, me on the other. We both loved it. Then back to Belfast City centre to buy our souvenirs. Our dinner was booked in one of the hotels. This day stayed with me for a few good reasons. The beauty we saw in the landscape, the Giant's Causeway, the funfair in Carrigfergus, and coming into Belfast on a bus with a Southern Ireland plate on the back.

Holy Mother of God, didn't the bus ahead of us blow up, just along the road we were travelling. The smell of smoke from the fire that was blazing from the blown-up bus and the smell of the petrol burning was choking us children. We were very lucky to be alive. Those children were also from the South, just like us. Innocent children, not much older than ourselves. That would have been our bus, only we got held up along the way with traffic, thank God. English squaddies and soldiers were everywhere we looked. We were all frightened when we saw them with their rifles in their arms.

The nuns tried to jolly us up by bringing us for our tea in a big hotel. All we really wanted was to go home fast to our Mammies and Daddies. We ate our sausage, egg, beans and chips, with bread and butter and a lovely cup of tea in a china cup and saucer. There were no complaints from the nuns because we all behaved. We were allowed go next door to a gift shop. I bought toffees and other trinkets. I wanted to buy my Daddy a box of sweets, but he was trying to lose weight. Yeah right, even I know drinking pints of porter doesn't help anyone lose weight. His belly was getting bigger instead of smaller.

Before we got back to Mount Sackville, my family had heard about the bomb on the television that Grandad had saved up for in the Credit Union. They all saw the bus going up in flames. Mam's heart was pumping with relief when she saw our bus coming up the road.

My Confirmation

I was very excited. It was coming near to my Confirmation Day, and Mam and I were kept busy, going in and out to the city on the No. 80 Luttrellstown bus. The happiness was really catching. I felt giddy and full of fun. We would check out Arnotts, Clerys and Dunnes. We traipsed around all the many rails. After a few weeks, Mam found her own outfit – the most beautiful tomato red two-piece suit, with a navy blue tie-style scarf to tie loosely around her neck. Holy God, Mam only bought herself a ginger-haired wig. Yes, honestly – it was hidden at the end of her shopping bag, out of sight. Why she bought this I do not know. We went into a smaller shop, and there was an amazing cream-coloured dress and coat, with a nice jockey hat to match. I tried them on. God I felt the bee's knees in my lovely rig-out. Mam loved it on me, too. She went off to pay for my rig-out. 'That's the two of us sorted,' Mam smiled and a pleased look came on her face.

A few weeks earlier I had got a grand pair of new brown leather shoes. In Clark's shoeshop they had the artificial crocodile design which was the latest fashion for children. They would look great after a good go with the shoe polish and a dry cloth.

Well, the hair was washed with Bristows 2-in-1 shampoo and conditioner on the morning of my Confirmation. Mam was very proud of my long curly hair. No one ever saw the torture it was getting those curls into my lovely hair, and the slaps I got on my legs – 'Will you stay blooming still.' Next minute, the sting of Mam's comb as she slapped me. Ah well, I did love the outcome of her hard work.

I had a fantastic new brown bag, my brown gloves, Confirmation medal and a little purse Nana Lizzy bought me to match the new stuff. Mam had me going around like a top model. I kept running into the bathroom to check how I looked. Yes, I liked what I saw. No cars were available to give us a lift, so we walked down to Chapelizod. Nana Lizzy was with us, but no sign of my Daddy! He left early that morning, and didn't mention anything about my Confirmation. This hurt Mam more than it hurt me. I was used to my Daddy ignoring me. I often wondered why he never bothered much about me, or what I had ever done to him.

Having practiced for months, I was ready for the Bishop to ask us all a question from the catechism about our religion. My tummy was doing its usual carry-on from nerves. All I was praying for was not to need a pee half-way through the morning. The Bishop put questions to a few children at the front. By the time he got to my row, it was simply a case of kissing the ring on his finger. Phew, thank God, I could relax a bit then.

We all met up outside the chapel in Chapelizod to have our photographs taken by our parents. Then into town to meet Aunt Sis in the pub. I got a professional photo done first in the photo shop in Mary Street. Then it was out to Myo's with Aunt Sis in tow. Holy God, why do I have to suffer so much? Why does bloody drink always ruin my lovely day? We met up with cousins twice removed on my Grandad's side. The reason they were distant was because when they left, my handbag with all my money was gone in their car! Never to be seen or got again... Mam and Nana tried their house, but no-one opened the door. They were peeping out from behind their curtains. We waved in at them. I had all my bits in that lovely bag. Mam had been delighted meeting these grand cousins of hers. No wonder they were wealthy, robbing young teenagers on their Confirmation Day. We ended up in the Angler's Rest pub; both Mam and Sis were in the divine horrors drunk.

Finally, home to the lodge and Nana asked me what was wrong. I burst into tears, telling her about my bag, prayer-book, purse and the money that I had collected all through my Confirmation Day, now all gone. Mammy didn't have a clue what was going on, and was completely out of it. They staggered up to our bedroom. I was put in the end of Mammy and Daddy's bed. Sis slept in mine; God bring on the morning please. The smell of drink from three boozed adults, plus Daddy and Mammy were at the karma sutra and there was me stuck in the end of the bed. I was afraid of my life to complain in case my Daddy burst me with a kick. He never liked me when he was drinking, which was his ongoing hobby. One thing's for sure, I'll never forget the big days in my life. The next morning found a few sick-looking heads at the breakfast table. Funny we never met those relations ever again.

Christmas Memories

I love Christmas in Ireland. To this day, Christmas brings a flame of love to my heart. It brings out the small child in me. All the razzmatazz of the beautifully decorated shops. Visiting old Santy and his little elves, plus Rudolf the red-nose reindeer and the lovely present coming away from the white-bearded Santy, who nearly always smelled like me Da did after a night in the boozer. Well at least Santy didn't fart, or if he did they were quiet ones and didn't stink like me Da's.

Every year the Guinness family would lay on a bus to take all the workers' children to the pantomime in the good old Gaiety, with the wonderful Maureen Potter, God bless her. As usual, no expense was spared for my clothes for the party. A beautiful velvet dress in navy blue, red or green would be purchased, or one of the older dresses brought to the dressmaker's house to be re-frilled and bowed in different coloured ribbon or buttons. It would look brand spanking new for me to wear with lovely new ribbons for my hair, new white socks and new Clark's shoes in the latest fashion – maybe patent leather crocodile or snakeskin shoes, or the odd fancy bow detail. I always got new knickers, vest, socks and cardigan for all these occasions.

Leaving the house with a fancy coat with a fur neckline, and imitation fur mittens, I would feel like a little princess, with my hair freshly washed with Bristow's shampoo and conditioner and my face and bits washed with Pear's soap. After that Mam would spend ages putting in my lovely ringlets, though I never liked the slaps I got, because I refused to keep quiet having to get those curling rags in my hair. My parents always kept me dressed very well, as best they could afford, even if they both liked their booze-filled weekends. I never remember ever going short of food, heat or home comforts.

On these Christmas outings, the Guinness family always hired the VIP box at the Gaiety Theatre. Sitting right up over the stage was lovely. We would all be up there looking down, to see if we knew anyone from Mount Sackville School in Knockmaroon, or the boys' school in Castleknock, to make faces at them from our VIP fancy box. At the interval, one of the helpers would bring in sweets to suck, crisps and Miwadi orange to quench our thirst and help us roar even louder 'He's behind ya!' in the second half of the pantomime. We would be hoarse going home on the coach from all the roaring at the pantomime performers.

We would be delighted to be allowed in to the big house to sing carols with her Ladyship and the children. We always joined in and the children were given lovely gifts before we left the mansion. There were great presents for each worker's child. This is where I got my copy of *Little House on the Prairie*, about a family named Ingalls. They were living out on the prairie in America. I never got the same story book twice; they must have kept a record of the books they had given me as a present. We were served afternoon tea with delicately cut ham and cucumber sandwiches, and tiny finger cakes for an extra treat. Then our parents would come about six to collect us. We always remembered to thank his Lordship and her Ladyship and the young Guinness family members for our lovely day out to the Gaiety Theatre. To this day, these happy memories stay with me, giving me hope for Christmas and each bright new year ahead. The child inside of each of us comes alive at this beautiful time of the year.

Getting Fruity with Tadpoles

I loved walking around the grounds of the main house. They had their own outdoor swimming-pool and beside it were four damson trees. At a certain time of the year, it would be laden with fine juicy damsons, ready for picking. Before I started to pick the fruit I always got into the pool. It was kept empty, except for a drop of rain water. There were lots of tadpoles. I would bring a jam jar with me to catch them and watch them swim around in the jar. There were a few little ponds further into the woods. The men in charge of the grounds made them for her Ladyship. Some of these ponds had different colour goldfish and were covered in beautiful water-lilies and green moss.

Mushrooms and Cowdung

It was lovely to go for walks with my Grandad Ned, and our two doggies, Lassie and Towser. I would always be tired coming home – Grandad would walk the legs off me. In August or September, we would pick wild mushrooms in the cow fields, on the way home from our nature walks. He would show me the right ones to pick. We would pick lots of them and when we got home, out came the butter. He would clean the mushrooms and see there were no worms after burrowing in through the stem. If not, they were put on the top of the Stanley range till they went brown, and the butter was melted on top. I would be in heaven, they tasted so lovely, washed down with a cup of Grandad's cha after our long walk.

There were times I had to pick cow dung for the fire. Ah God, I hated this job. It had to be good hard old cow shite. Grandad would make me take off my shoes and socks, go into the cow field, and find the big cow pats. I then had to put my bare foot in it to see if it was hard. Sometimes the cowpats were only hard on top, and the poo would ooze up through my toes. 'Jaysus Elizabeth child, the look of disgust on your puss was priceless', Grandad always said. He would try hard not to laugh.

I hated doing this awful task, but the dried cow poo kept great heat in our fire in the night time. There were also loads of 'cogs' (cones) from the fir trees, and fallen branches. Before the TB, Grandad, Neddy, and my Dad Algy would spend a few nights cutting big trees over in the wood and carrying them home to keep us all warm in the winter months. Now I was gathering cow poo and cogs and twigs – a big come down in the lodge!

My Hammering Heart

One windy, damp and dark Wednesday October night, as I lay in bed listening to the big copper beech tree branches hitting the tiles on the roof, the rain constantly pelting on our bedroom window, watching the embers flickering in the remains of the sparse fire, wishing and praying sleep would come, I tossed and turned, knowing something was up with my Mam. She lay all crouched up and groaning in the double bed. I knew that Daddy wasn't in bed yet, as there was no smell of stale beer and wind. As a rule, my mother always stayed up to heat and dish up Daddy's evening meal and have the chat about comings and goings of the locality, no matter how late it got, especially after my Daddy spending a long tiring day on his feet at some farm or race course.

This night in particular, me Ma didn't seem herself. She called me over to whisper in my ear, to stop anyone hearing her. Downstairs, they were glued to the evening news on the black and white telly. Anyway I ran into the toilet and got the pofer, as Grandad called my potty. Janey Mack, I hated trying to sneak the potty up to bed; the minute Grandad spotted it under my arm or hidden behind my back, the teasing would start and at times I would feel like bawling my eyes out. Oh, the embarrassment of having a potty!

The time my mother bought this new potty, she also bought a brown fluffy flower design mat at a sale in Arnotts. Nice and posh it was, and it went well in front of the fire in our bedroom. It felt great, us both sitting on the mat with the lights out, the flickering flames lighting up the walls and ceiling. Our small fire only needed to be lit on blustery or frosty winter nights. We would have fantastic fun making shadow animals using our hands and fingers. Then Mam or I had to guess what animal it was. God, the craic brought tears of joy to my tired eyes. We would sit on the fluffy mat by the fire, and Mam would end the fun with night stories as I got cosy in my bed. She would start telling me ghostie stories and I would be afraid of my life. I loved her telling me the long and short tales about Ma's own childhood days, though, her awesome tales from years ago.

Well, like I was saying, tonight, for some reason, I got this unusual feeling in my belly before coming upstairs to bed. Mam was after whispering to me, 'We're going to have a nice relaxing night. I'm going to bed, Elizabeth child. Say goodnight to Nana and Grandad, get your potty and we will head to bed, pet' rubbing my mass of curly auburn hair.

There must have been something really wrong, as Ma turned the big light out immediately. She had lit the fire in our room earlier than usual. We went straight into our beds. No making animal fingers and having a laugh in front of our fire tonight, or her teaching me my lessons, counting a few numbers extra every night, or how to spell complicated words like Constantinople or Mississippi. Eventually I dozed off to a fitful sleep.

When I awoke in the morning, my Dad had gone off to his day job. Ma was out of the bed, bawling crying, and a stream of blood was coming away from her from below. When I saw the blood I thought 'Jaysus me poor Ma is going to die on me.' My heart was hammering like the devil inside my small rib cage. It was banging like billyo, sounding like a machine gun on reload. It felt like it was going to pop out my two ears. I was gone to the stage of nearly hysterical with the terrible fright. 'Ah God, help us quick.'

Well God really must have heard my prayer because I heard Nana Lizzy shifting for work. I wanted nothing better than to yell 'Nana come quick. Ma's dying on us.' With that Mam put her hand across my mouth saying, 'Shhhhhh now child, it's okay. I'm alright, Elizabeth. Quiet now girly, please. We don't want to alarm your Nana Lizzy now do we.' I felt like saying 'What about me? I'm nearly shitting myself here.' Ah to hell with this, I thought – 'Nana, quick, Ma's not well'. Well, be jeepers if looks could kill, my Ma would be burying me with a hatchet. 'If she doesn't die on me first!', I was thinking in my own childish mind.

Nana came in like a bolt of lightning into our bedroom. 'Louie, Lou what's up?' They sent me down the stairs for something or other. I heard whispering – adult talk they called it. Not for young ears, I was told. I came back up the stairs, two at a time. 'Elizabeth, help your Ma. Please go to the drawer and get some more bath towels, quickly now child.' Nana got the hot water, Dettol, the wash stuff – Pears soap and the flannel – plus these funny looking towels me Ma hid in her drawer where her nighties were kept. Ma cleaned herself up and told me, 'Now girlie keep this to yourself, it's our secret. The least anyone knows the better.'

They kept me off school on this terrifying day. We had a bowl of lovely warm Ready Brek with lashings of sugar on it and a nice hot cup of sugary tea – a treat to try and bring me around after the fright. When our local Castleknock Village doctor arrived, it was me who got his water bowl ready to wash his hands. He was a lovely, gentle, caring, understanding doctor. Nana Lizzy was going off to work after cleaning everything up in our room and changing the sheets on me Ma's bed so Dr Nelson could check her out properly up in the bedroom for privacy.

I was listening at the bedroom door. He asked Ma to go into the Mater Hospital for a few days.

'Oh God no, Doctor Nelson, I'm far too busy. I'm needed here, the child, my husband, Daddy and Mammy. They all need me.'

'Now Louise you have yourself to care for in this situation first and foremost. They will all cope well enough without you, Louise. For a few days woman. You need a transfusion after losing so much blood'.

My Ma replied, 'Oh no Doctor, I'm not going in. I might not come out again.'

'Okay, I will give you iron tablets to help you. Take them daily. Please come to my surgery soon, now, Louise.'

Ma told him politely, 'I'm fine and thank you for coming, Doctor,' as she paid his consultation fee. I heard noise and scarpered quickly and quietly down the stairs, before I got caught being brazen and disobeying me Ma. I sat at the table looking all innocent, pretending to be intent on colouring with crayons on a colouring book. Oh Janey Mack, that had made me worse. That's always the way – nosing and prying doesn't pay dividends to bold children. They told me not to come up the stairs and I didn't listen. I remember it like it's all going on in my mind still.

To say me Ma was very quiet for weeks after this would be an understatement. I missed the stories and counting lessons big time. Everyone in our house noticed the difference in Ma, how pale and quiet she was, but she just passed it off as needing a tonic and the doctor having her on iron tablets to build her up after the cold winter. 'Summer's coming and I will be grand when I get a bit of sun on my face and bones,' was her answer every time someone mentioned how ill she looked. God bless her heart. Unknown to anyone only Doctor Nelson, Nana Lizzy and me, Ma had lost an embryo baby, and it was a great wrench to her, as she really wanted this baby. It was in later years I learned all this about her miscarriage. Sure, I thought me Ma was really going to die on us that horrid morning, right there in front of me two brown eyes.

OMG I'm Heartbroken

The months trailed on, winter turned to spring, and then summer time arrived. With it came the holiday crowd. In June came Aunt Betty's sister on holiday from England. In tow was her husband, Uncle Patrick or Pat for short – a cool cockney barrow boy when he was younger, full of the cockney rhyming slang. They use this lingo in the east end of London. They say if a cockney is not born near the Church of Mary

Le Bow, then they're not true cockneys. His family had been moved to a Wiltshire town named Swindon. My Aunt Betty lived and worked in this town. They met, fell in love and yeah that makes Pat me Uncle. God, I couldn't understand a word. It was double Dutch to me. They brought their son Brian, ten and half years old; I was just gone eleven.

I was sorry they showed up out of the blooming blue at all, because it brought the worst news ever. My whole world fell apart. Mam was going over to live with one of her sisters in Swindon, Wiltshire. Holy Jaysus, what am I going to do? Will I go with her, and pray we would come back home again? Or stay in Knockmaroon Lodge and live unhappily without my dear Mother?

Mam won, hands down. Besides, I was sure it was going to be just an extra long holiday, and we would definitely come back home again. I thought she was trying to frighten my Dad. I'm sure the reason they split up was because I was growing into a teenager – eleven years old – and it was not right to be sleeping in their room. They had no proper privacy for themselves. Ma kept on asking Dad to find a house for us. He never got around to it. He didn't have time. It was always put on the long finger. 'I will do it tomorrow, next week, next month, Louie'. It was on the never never list. She gave up hope and headed off to pastures new to make a life for us both. Mind you, I'm sure the booze didn't help matters for them. It's a curse in many relationships, and can break up the best of families. A sad fact. If Dad had loved us, I'm sure he would have come after us. Too fond of the dreaded auld drink, and his cronies, as Mam called Daddy's friends and work colleagues.

Jeepers, I was gutted. It felt very strange and unreal to me as an eleven-year old child, saying goodbye to both my faithful dogs Lassie and Towser, my favourite playmate and loyal pet. That dog never failed to sit waiting for me every single day at the front door, with his lead in his mouth, wagging his tail like mad the minute he heard me coming in the gate. I would push open the front door and he would jump up on me with great excitement. To this day I can remember the joy and happiness Towser brought me. Even after I left for England, that old faithful still waited without fail, sitting waiting and I never came to see him after school each day. Aw God, my heart was breaking. Why, dear God?

I ran out to see Lassie, and feed the chickens and collect the eggs, before it was time to leave for the airport. I gave hugs to Grandad, Nana, Nedser and Patty. As usual, my Dad was nowhere to be seen. Before we left the house, I ran up to our bedroom one more time, just for a last quick look. My heart was racing; I had a strong urge to look out the upstairs window. Jaysus there he was, my Dad half scuttered, I'm sure. I shouted down 'Goodbye Daddy'. He had the sneaky hip flask in his hand and was after swigging a big gulp from it. He looked up at me, tears in his eyes.

'Fuck off you little bitch, you're worse than the other whore,' he shouted up at me. 'You're well fucking matched, the two of you'.

Well, his last words broke my heart in two. I would live with this forever. I wasn't even sure what that bad word was, but I knew it wasn't a very nice thing to say to me. I had a lump in my throat and a desperate pain in my gut. The tears rolled down my cheeks in torrents. Christ, I was sorry I went up the fecking stairs at all. We took off in the taxi that was ordered. I left the only home I ever knew for whatever lay ahead.

'Oh God,' I thought, 'I have far more to go.'

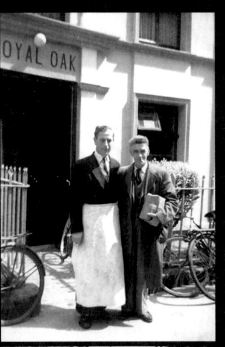
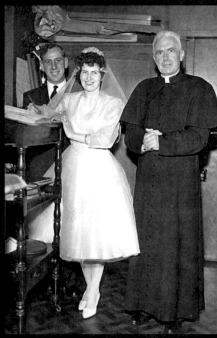
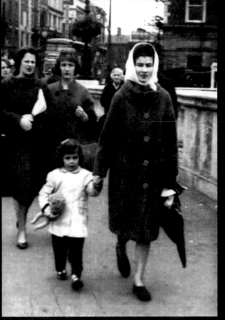
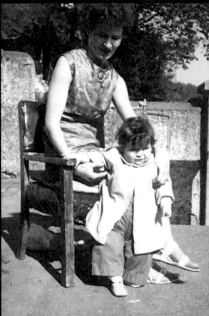

Clockwise from top left: My Daddy, Algy McCue and a local man he knew.
Mammy and Daddy's wedding.   Aw, bless, Ma and me. She adored her sickly tot Elizabeth Ann.
Lizzy and Louie, O'Connell Bridge.

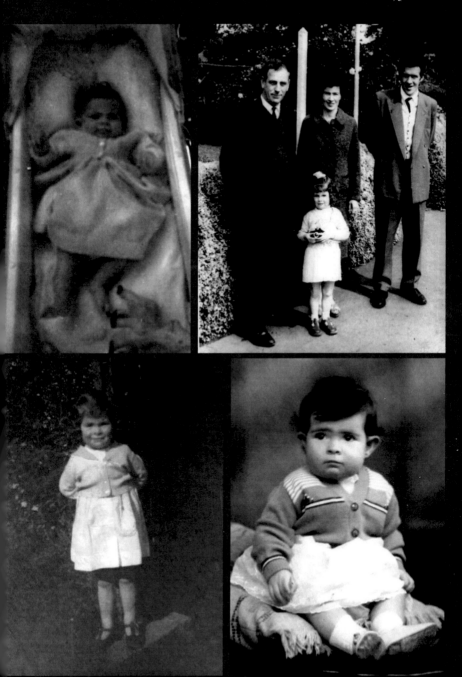

Clockwise from top left: Little me in my pram. Daddy, Mammy, Nedser and me.
Thursday's Child. Little me, about two years old.

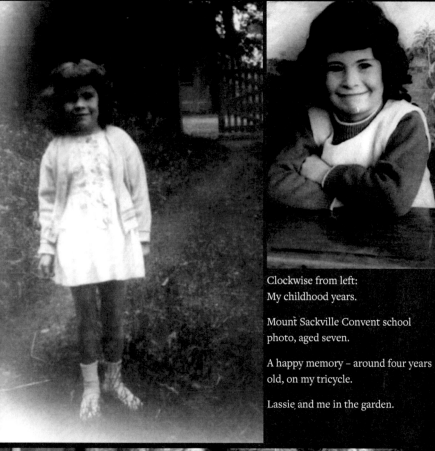

Clockwise from left:
My childhood years.

Mount Sackville Convent school
photo, aged seven.

A happy memory – around four years
old, on my tricycle.

Lassie and me in the garden.

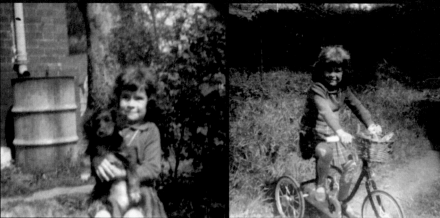

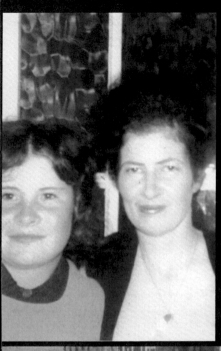

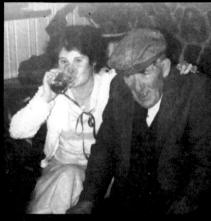

Clockwise from left:

Liz (11) and Louie after arriving in Swindon 1971.

Grandad Ned and me on the lash in Myo's Pub.

Barney D, my dear Mam and my pride and joy, Gemma, enjoying the sunshine.

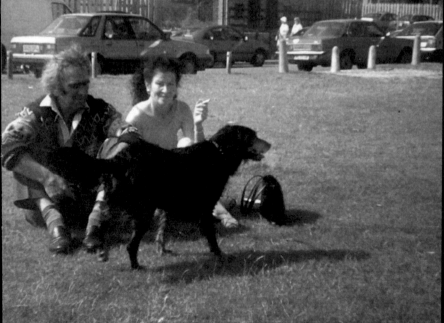

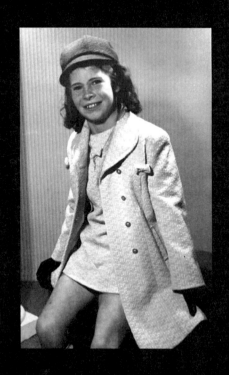

Part Three

Rude Awakening: Troubled Teenage Years of an Irish Emigrant

The plane took off. I was sitting heartbroken beside my eleven-year-old cousin Brian. He looked like a girl, with his big head of blond curly hair. I liked him really. Just not today. Ma sat on the end seat, Betty on the next aisle, with her husband Pat. Because I was looking for anyone to blame except my own Mam and Dad, and not knowing my Uncle Pat that well, he got the brunt of the anger that was deep inside my heart.

'We're off on our new adventure, Elizabeth. Are you excited child?' Mam enquired, waiting patiently for my reply. In my own mind I was thinking, 'I am not!' It felt like my heart and soul had been ripped out of my body. I felt like I was slowly dying deep inside my heart. 'Ah yeah Ma, I'm excited,' I answered, thinking to myself, 'I will play along with her stupid game, just for the hell of it. Nothing ventured, nothing gained,' a brazen head on me. 'I will pretend I'm on my holidays. I have my fingers, legs, toes, even me two bleeding eyes crossed.'

'Please God, bring us home very soon. Don't forsake me, God. Amen,' was my constant prayer all through the flight. 'I'm not one bit happy. Aw God, life is not flipping fair.' I felt like bawling me eyes out, but I knew if I started I wouldn't stop until all my tears ran free, and that would take forever.

New surroundings. Going to an English school. Trying to make new friends. The way they talked. It all felt strange to me at the tender young age of twelve.

We moved in with Aunt Bridget, her Polish husband and their six children: three boys and three girls. They were lovely to us. It was only their Daddy that always frightened the bejesus out of me. There was no food wastage allowed in the house. Even the mangy crust on the bread, that I hated, had to be eaten, even stale or dried up or out of date. All kids' plates had to leave the table empty. It all had to be eaten, and if I threw the crust under the table, he made me get down on my hands and knees, pick that up off the floor, and eat it. Ah Jeepers, I would be gagging and my tummy would do turnovers.

To me he was an awful man, not knowing he was from a concentration camp, or what a Nazi concentration camp even was. I never realised what he truly suffered in his younger Polish years. The time of Hitler, my uncle was put in the concentration camp at Auschwitz.

I was glad when Aunt Betty and Uncle cock-sparrow Pat, and my young cousin Brian took us into their house, out of pity for us, mostly. We were like waifs and bloody strays, shifting from Biddy to Betty. No sooner had we moved in there than Ma took to the drink again. She was after meeting another Plastic Paddy, as the Irish people overseas are sometimes called. A new man. After that I never saw much of her, between her working in Garrard's factory by day, and going to the pub with her quare fella all evening long, then back with him to his latest digs. We always called this new man, Frank, 'the quare fella'.

Mam had a bun in the oven, I was told. Now I didn't know why she had a bun in the oven, or whose oven. We only had Aunty Betty and Uncle Pat's oven, and there was definitely no bun in there. 'I keep on looking,' I would tell the school kids that taunted me. It was only later I learned that the English saying meant someone was pregnant. A good few months later, on my fourteenth birthday – Sunday March 10, 1974 – Ma gave birth to my sister. Anna-Maria, she named her. When she finally brought Anna home I thought how beautiful this little baby was.

Yes I was jealous, but I did love the child in my own way. Not that I ever showed baby Anna-Maria this, and at times was very unkind. To this day I dislike myself for this action. If I could, then I sure as hell would turn back the clock.

I wasn't brought to the hospital to see my baby sister when she arrived. This made me feel unloved and unwanted, just a lost cause. Goodness, the house was very crowded! Everyone got on reasonably okay, bar the odd scrap between us two cousins. Brian and me wanted the job of going to the chippy on a Thursday, which was pay night for the adults. One of us was always sent around to get the Thursday treat of fish and chips, and burgers for us children. We both knew whoever went could spend three pound on sweets and minerals. It was a great trial to get the job of going – we would both be black and blue with bruises, and chunks of hair missing. We loved each other really. Sweets always bonded us. They never realised why Brian and me would kick one another, and pull each other's hair. I was even known to bite him. If he went and I didn't, there would be merry hell to pay. Betty sent Uncle Pat around one evening for the supper to teach us a lesson for fighting every week. He came back and he gave out to us both for being brazen, for not bringing home the correct change. That put an end to our Thursday night treats in Mr Rose's shop in Cavendish Square!

Betty was later to get a bun in her own oven – her baby son John was born seven months after Anna-Maria, in November '74. Eventually we got called for our own council house in Rodbourne, which is near Swindon town centre. We got settled in and were getting on grand, doing a bit of painting and extra cleaning. The only trouble was, money was hard to find with two children and no one working. We made do and got by, though. It bonded us a bit more, I think.

Often at night I would lay in bed, tossing and turning, my tummy gurgling with dreaded wind pain. This was due to the heaps of vegetables Ma put in our five day stew. We called it Ethiopian stew, because it would never make us fat. Each Saturday Ma would buy a half pound of beef, cut in pieces. To this she added as much vegetables and potatoes that she could find in the cupboard. This kept us going for days, with sliced bread and cheap margarine. My God, the 'wind' blowing through our house was brutal. A gas mask was a priority on my next Christmas wishlist! That and Motilium tablets. Still, it was better than starving. We were embarrassed when family or friends came to visit. We never had a biscuit to offer with their cup of tea and tinned condensed milk. We used this in our tea every day. The visitors often refused tea after their first cup. To this day, even thinking about this tinned milk makes me gag.

Aw, Ma did her best to fill our hungry bellies with the money from the Department of Social Security. After paying her weekly bills, and getting a few necessary items for baby Anna-Maria, there wasn't much left for food. It felt strange, because at home in Knockmaroon the food put on the table was plentiful, nourishing and very filling. A stew made for the Smith family, we could nearly walk on it. The meat was plentiful and tasty, and the juices were thick, unlike Swindon stew!

But it was too late to go home to Ireland now. Daddy had left the lodge and gone to live with his sister Carmel near Dublin. Carmel's husband Mick had died from a massive heart attack, God rest him. He was a fine man who adored me. Plus, Ma had a little baby in tow. This wouldn't look good: Grandad Ned and Nana Lizzy would find this too much of a scandal to bear, listening to the gossips in the community.

Everyone knew Louise and Albert had split up. Ma went to a solicitor in Swindon to end the marriage. Lawyers tried to serve divorce papers on my Daddy, but Grandad sent the letter back to England unopened. Divorce was not legal in Ireland. Perhaps Ma thought the quare fella, Frank, would marry her, since she had his baby in her arms. But I bet my Daddy would have welcomed us back, no matter what, because he loved his wife Louie dearly. Mam was too smitten with my baby sister Anna-Maria and Frank, though.

For all the good he seemed to me – the quare fella was often in 'her Majesty's service', in Bristol, Avon. Frank was a devil for driving fast cars. He thought that all he had to do was buy an old banger car, get in, and drive like a mad yoke around the streets of Swindon with no tax, driving licence, insurance or MOT! The police would often catch him coming up to the full moon. For some reason Frank and the full moon had a rendezvous together; it brought out the blackguarding in him. Nine times out of ten he would get a holiday in HMP – Her Majesty's Prison. Bed and full board!

Frank suffered terribly with his nerves; it later turned out he had bipolar disorder. He couldn't help his high jinxes.

I remember when Frank was due out Ma went all gooey-eyed, like a blooming teenager. Playing the same record, over and over, 'Tie a Yellow Ribbon Round the Old Oak Tree' sung by Tony Orlando. There was Frank languishing in the nick, with three good meals a day and as much real milk as he could drink in his tea. No pains in his belly from Ethiopian food like us, no bills or household worries like trying to file down old brown pennies to fit in our electric meter. We hated the dark cold nights because we had no coal for the fire or any type of heating to keep us or baby Anna warm. If it was brutally cold, there would be nothing for it only going to bed early.

A man that Ma knew undid the lock on our meter for us. That was great, because we had free electric and free heating. We saved a few bob to buy a cheap, second-hand electric heater. Fantastic! At last, we felt like there was a God up there. We would leave the oven on at night and sit out in the kitchen, chatting and planning our goals. It was a smaller room to heat. Now we knew this was against the law, but God knew we were desperate at this time.

Frank arrived to live with us in Rodbourne Road. This didn't go down well with me or him. We were like alternators ready to explode whenever our wires connected together. He wasn't there long with us, and everything quietened down again. It was rumoured he was in Liverpool, but no one knew. Still, we were used to not having a man around the house.

One evening Aunty Betty and Pat's friend Sean called with an urgent message. Mam's mother, my Nana Lizzy, was dying of cancer, and she hadn't long to go – a matter of weeks, if that. There was still no sign of Frankie; I knew he wasn't in Liverpool: he was on his extended holiday. At first I was to go and stay with my cousin Helen, who I loved. We got on well. She was married to Tommy; they had one baby girl, a pretty child named Sammy for short. There were only a few months between Sammy, Anna and Betty's baby John. Betty was now pregnant again, not long after having baby John. It was unadvisable to travel being so near to the birth, only two weeks. How strange, both at the same time: Aunty Betty having baby number two, and dear Nana going to die. To me, in my 15 year old eyes, life was right quare.

Bridget would pay to bring me back to Knockmaroon Lodge for Nana's funeral, instead of my staying with my cousin Helen. Mam and me travelled by plane to Dublin to spend the last weeks with her Mam and my dear Nana Lizzy. I adored every bone in that dear woman's body, God bless her. Seemingly Nana wanted to see me – her dear Elizabeth: 'Where's the child, Ned? I want to see the child.' And so it was arranged I would come home. Nana was not dying without telling me she loved me, and she managed to whisper it many times as I lay comfortably beside her in the double bed. The pain she must have been in, but Nana waited for us all to arrive home from Swindon. All but Betty, her daughter, due to give birth.

A few days later they started to up her pain relief drug, Morphine, a bit more each day. I tried not to cry, honestly I did. But I couldn't help it. My throat would start contracting and the tears would be ready to flow. This meant I wasn't allowed up to Nana Lizzy's bedroom. I heard my Grandad saying 'Don't be letting Elizabeth up them stairs, Louie.' They all thought Nana didn't know she was dying; you can bet my beautiful Nana Lizzy knew well. There was no pulling the wool over Lizzy Smith's mystic eyes. She was too cute: a very intuitive woman. Nothing or no-one got one over on Nana Lizzy Smith.

The day I stopped going up to the bedroom to spend time with her, that was the start of the countdown to her passing. They all said she called for Elizabeth a few times before she passed over. We were never sure if Nana Lizzy was calling her daughter Betty, or me. In my eyes, it was me she wanted because I was her little star, but I say that only because she didn't really know her other wonderful grandchildren that well. They lived in the Shires of England, all but my cousin Michelle who was far too small to be by Nana's side as she lay dying. There were ten years between us in age, but Michelle and myself, we were close to our dear Nana Lizzy.

I often wrote long essay-style letters from England. These letters were sent home religiously to my dear Nana and Grandad, and Uncle Neddy RIP. I loved them both very dearly, my Nana and Grandad Ned. It hurt my heart being held captive in England. Well, that's how it felt to me at the time. My heart ached for my old homestead. This was where I truly belonged, in Knockmaroon, County Dublin with my family, my dad Albert. I missed everyone terribly. I always felt really homesick living over in England when all I wanted was to be here. I remember we walked miles together, Nana and me, when I lived in the lodge with the family. We never stopped chatting about everything.

One time before we left for England, Nana woke up one morning in a desperate state. 'Neddy, where's Neddy. I dreamt he was dead.' She described the death in great detail, down to the marks and burns on his face and hands. Years later, in 1983, that exact accident happened, leaving the same markings on his body. Our Nedser died at the exact spot she predicted. We often laughed after the fright she gave us that morning, but we got a real fright when Neddy died as predicted. Only a mother knows. Nana Lizzy was my beautiful Earth angel, now my heavenly angel.

For the funeral, it was decided I would stay up in Aunty Patty and Uncle Dave's house, and mind little Michelle. They lived near enough to the lodge, up in Clonsilla. I didn't like that idea, but we stayed at home in the house until after Nana's burial, as Michelle was far too little at six years old, and I was going on 16 myself.

Grandad thought it might be a good idea to keep me living at home with them – to stay in Ireland and look after him and Neddy. My Ma wasn't having that: 'Aw no Daddy, Elizabeth has her exams and will be doing her GCE in July.' Well God forgive you Mammy, what a porker to tell my grandfather! I hardly ever went to school, and Mam knew this well. Most mornings we had no money for my school bus.

Before we left Ireland, I celebrated my sixteenth birthday in Knockmaroon. Even though it wasn't till March 10, Neddy, Grandad, and Patty all gave me money for a shopping trip to Penneys with Mam and Bridget. I bought new boots and a rig-out to wear. My Daddy called to see us in the lodge and wished me a very happy birthday. He took us both to Larry O'Byrne's pub for old time's sake. In the Angler's Rest there was ballroom dancing that night. Even though my Nana was gone to heaven it didn't feel wrong to be dancing. I even had a quiet glass of Babycham that my Daddy got me for my birthday. The two of them were doing a tango – Mam and Dad certainly knew their dance moves. We had to leave early, as Dad had to catch the last bus home. I spent a lovely evening with my dear parents. I never remember my Daddy giving me a hug, or telling me 'I love you chicken.' Chicken was his pet name for me.

Before I left Ireland I had to go to see Dr Nelson, our old general practitioner in the village. He prescribed me antibiotics for another kidney infection, a bad one this time. My kidneys were leaking protein, plus I had a horrible dose of cystitis in my bladder. A bad sign, Doctor Nelson was telling my mother.

A couple of days later we headed back to England, to our new home in Rodbourne Road. Bridget thought my Dad would give her my fare, after her paying to take me home. Mam couldn't afford to buy my ticket as well as her own, and Daddy always sent my Mam money, every single week without fail, for all the years I was at school. This was very good of my father.

I think the reason they split up was because I was growing into a teenager. I was twelve years old – it was not right to be sleeping in their bedroom with them. They had no privacy; they couldn't even chat without someone listening to their every word, both downstairs and up. Ma kept on asking my Dad to find us a house where we could be a proper family. It's an awful pity Daddy never got around to it; He would always put everything on the long finger, even though Ma told him she would leave him if he didn't cop himself on. 'I will do it tomorrow Louie, sure I never got round to it, chicken,' was always the answer. Louie got fed up and gave up hope, heading off to make a life for us both across the sea.

Mind you, I'm sure the booze didn't help matters. It's a curse in all relationships; it causes many breakups to the best of families. A sad fact. I always thought if my Daddy had loved us, he would have come after us. It's the drink and his cronies, as Ma would say. Drink makes people do quare things. It has a strong pull on the addict. It never helped with my dear father being a barman all his life. I now know the drink was his downfall. He loved us with all his heart, but he needed his booze much more than the love of his beautiful family. How sad a fact is this, dear readers?

The three of us flew out from Dublin to Bristol, all deep in our own sad thoughts. Sometimes things are best left unsaid. It took me a very long time to get over my Nana. I felt like I was going through all the stress and grief of moving to England again. At times it feels like my life is a rollercoaster, with more downs than ups.

The Wretched School Bullies

St Joseph's Comprehensive School, Swindon. Jaysus I hated that school! The bullies drove me mad with rage at times. They picked on me daily. I wasn't like them: I spoke and acted differently. One day not long after I started, the bullies tried to flush my head down the toilet bowl. I was petrified and in a state of shock and horror. My tears fell all that day. It took ages to forget those little wretches. My cousin Helen's neighbour, Anna, a big girl of fourteen, always stood up for me. Anna chased them off and threatened to give them all a beating, her and her four friends, all big girls. The bullies never repeated that trick on me again. Scallywags! I didn't go to school many days, if at all, from the age of fifteen. I disliked the place, and the pompous teachers. We never saw eye to eye. Some of the lessons bored me. After learning all my Irish history, then having to learn the English version from scratch... How ridiculous was that to a child? I truly hated school with a vengeance, and especially the bully bashers and gang leaders. Then there were follow-the-leader kids – they all wanted to be accepted into the gang. They didn't want to feel left out, or sent to Coventry as it was called in England when one was ousted from the group and the other children were not allowed to speak to them.

I was always out in the cold. Peculiar was my Nickname. McCue being my last name made it sound cute – Peculiar McCue. They got a good laugh on my account, the scrag heads. I became the peculiar one. I never spoke much in class, or to the rest of the girls or boys. The minute I opened my mouth they would tease the life out of me with their stupidity. 'Come on Doggie'. 'Here's the peculiar dog coming'. This because I would follow them around and just sit and listen to their fun when they were out playing with their friends after school.

They never realised the damage they did to my self-esteem. I was in bits every single night. I went home to comfort-eat a whole loaf of bread with butter and jam. This was when we lived with my Aunt Betty in their house. She would be very cross when the bread for Uncle Pat's lunch was gone. He worked nights in a factory. Brian or myself would have to run and buy another loaf of bread for the evening. I'm sure Betty thought we both had ringworms, as my cousin was as bad as me for food bingeing. But cousin Brian was very lucky, being thin and gangly. I started to blow up to nearly 11 stone.

Because I always had kidney infections, I had a great excuse not to attend school much. I eventually refused to go in at all or if I did, it was just to sign the register in the morning. The teachers didn't care at all. I wasn't worth their time or effort. Yet I really wanted to be accepted by them all. After all, it wasn't my fault my Ma and Daddy didn't get on together, and I was brought almost kicking and ranting over to the shires of England. The nuns in Mount Sackville were far more tender than the teachers in St Joe's in Swindon, that's for sure.

There was a job advertised in the Evening Advertiser, looking for a young and vibrant silver service waitress to work full-time on a temporary basis to see if the candidate was suitable for the job at the Goddard Arms, Old Town, Swindon.

A Pony with a Big Kick

Spring of 1976. I was 16 years old, almost ready to leave school – only two weeks until I could officially leave. This certainly pleased me. Thank God the damn torture was over. 'I have done my penance,' I thought. No more of my head getting pushed down the smelly toilet bowl, and the little rips threatening to flush it if I refused to give them my dinner ticket or the lunch money I had in my pocket.

The years at school in England had made me prone to self-harm by cutting my skin with any sharp object I could possibly get my hands on. If I could cut myself it released my anger and the pain eased. I felt at peace, a warmth came over my body. It never lasted long.

Next, I started to starve my body of nutrients. Or binge-eat and then make myself really sick by drinking a couple of pints of water. If that didn't work, I would roll up pieces of toilet roll paper and stick it down my throat to make me gag. There would be tears streaming down my cheeks from hurting myself. I knew it was wrong, but I couldn't help this sad retaliation on my body. I hated eating in case I got fat again. I was like a walking skeleton. It was like there were no lights on in the attic, my Mam said. I had lost all emotion. I would walk miles on end, and do about two hundred sit ups, until my tummy and sides hurt badly from the strain of over-exercising. This was my control. I had nothing, but by doing all this abuse to myself, I felt great inside mentally.

Subconsciously I was a complete mess. My Nana was dead. That certainly didn't help matters; I was grieving. The kids at school wrecked my head with their constant put downs. Mam had no time for me for many years, really since we left our home in Castleknock. My Daddy didn't love me, or so I thought, thanks to his cruel words before we left the lodge for England.

I felt like I was on top of the world; lack of food and the body being deprived of nutrients and minerals were causing lack of oxygen and low energy. It brought on an unreal out of body experience. I had a feeling of liberation, like I was floating on air. Weird and warped as this might seem to some, this was my only power, or maybe I only thought this because I was far too scared to change this antagonistic abuse on my fragile body and mind. To people who have never walked a gruesome path in life like this, it must seem very strange indeed. What I felt was power and self-control, although I was killing myself, body, soul and mind.

The Goddard Arms

At 17, I had my job in the Goddard Arms in Old Town, and I also got taken on as a bar person in a local pub near my home in Swindon. The men that normally drank in this pub were hard-working Irish navvies. They liked their few pints after a heavy day on the building sites. The men usually got out of their work van and straight into the pub around six-thirty in the evening. They would still be there when the bell for last orders rang. There would be the occasional fight brewing for weeks between the men of different counties.

I lied about my age so the landlord would employ me. It was 'cash-in-hand'. I sometimes worked seven nights a week for a few hours, from seven in the evening until whatever time the clientele would stagger out the back door or up the stairs to their beds. The pub was a rundown hotel and had rooms upstairs. This meant the landlady would do bed and breakfast for the English men that were working in

Swindon. They travelled down from Coventry and Grimsby or other faraway places. The Irish men would stay in the locality, in houses that had rooms especially for them.

Saturdays were always hectic. Sometimes the man of the house or his son might try it on with me. This repulsed me. My tummy would heave. The father was large with very receding hair – not very pleasing to the eye. Because his Dad was paying me, the young lad also thought he could get his money's worth. Well, the least told about this side of things, the less embarrassing for all concerned.

How I kept the two jobs going is beyond me, but I needed the money because I was getting a need for whatever alcohol would numb my mind. A drink called Pony, in a little bottle, was a great one for me – I didn't need much money to blot my mind out. After the pub shut, I was to take a double brandy from whatever patrons were staying in the pub for a 'lock-in'. I wasn't to drink this drink but put the money in the till for the landlord. To hell with that! 'Down the hatch Lizzy,' I'd say as I knocked the drink back. 'Way hay, up yours landlord', I would be thinking to the flabby old git that owned the pub. I just didn't give a shite about any of them. His wife had left the landlord years before, fed up of being used and abused. He next had a Scottish woman with him. She was lovely, but not very streetwise, and she really just didn't know what was going on under her own nose. This woman got terminal cancer and died, God rest her dear soul.

The dreaded drink would burst the head off me the next morning when I had to get up for my silver service waitress work in the posh hotel in Old Town. I was getting very bony and anorexic. If I ate anything, I would feel guilty for overeating, and then I would run out to the toilet and puke my guts up. I would fill myself with fluid and this made it easier to vomit. It was a self-defeating cycle: the little child trapped inside my soul was taking an awful bashing from the manic depressive teenager that I was now.

When I was ready for work in the morning, I had to look in my Ma's big wardrobe mirror to see if I looked okay. I did this every single morning before getting into the taxi. The manic monkey voice would start its egoistic abusive put-downs in my mind: 'Look at the state of you, you big fat ugly thing. Who would want you? You're a horrid looking girl.' The more my inner voice attacked me, the worse my eating and boozing got. 'Jesus Lizzy, you're going to destroy your body and mind girl,' Mam would often say. As soon as I was home and ate the supper cooked for me, it was the same scenario: upstairs to the toilet, away from prying eyes or hearing ears.

After the vomiting, I would get myself ready and head off to the pub. This was in all weathers, every evening. If I wasn't working, it made no difference: I had to go down the pub where the drink would flow for me, somehow or other. At times I wouldn't come home. The taxi would arrive at quarter to seven in the morning but no Elizabeth was to be found in the house. My late arrival in the morning would throw everyone in the hotel kitchen out of kilter. Chef would be very cross with me. This went on until my body really gave me big problems.

My kidneys were giving up, with the acid-reflux, ulcers and heartburn from all the acid in the vomit. At times the pain would be excruciating. The brandy would bring even more hell on my body. I was coming up to nineteen years of age, but my body was giving up. I couldn't eat, even if I needed to. By now my kidneys didn't work very well at all. My hair started to fall out, which was even worse than when I had kept pulling out clumps from my sore scalp – another form of self-abuse.

Eventually I was called to the manager's office in the Goddard Arms Hotel. A series of problems had been recorded in the workbook – arriving late or leaving early. My appearance didn't help matters. We had a strict rule of clean nails, hair and good manners at all times, but now my hair looked straggly due to vitamin and mineral deficiencies. I wore a scarf at night in the pub but this was most certainly not allowed in my day job, and my nails were often painted. Nor was the manager pleased with my behaviour or language following an evening knocking back bottles of Pony in the pub.

He was very nice to me, though. 'Go home Elizabeth and think about your life,' he said. He told me to decide what I wanted for myself and then, if I got my act together, come back and speak to him.

God, was I afraid to go home and tell my own mother I was laid off work! The first thing I did was go to the Wimpy Bar in the town centre and order myself a meal. I asked the Turkish man that owned it if he had any jobs going. Luckily he had one starting on the following Monday as a Wimpy waitress, washer up and dog's body. Well, it was a job, with money coming in for my keep. I met a guy I knew and headed off on the booze.

Well Mam went ballistic, roaring and shouting at me when I eventually got home. 'You couldn't even be bothered to come home and tell me the manager let you go. Oh no, only your Aunt Biddy told me you were gone, I wouldn't have even known about it.'

The job in the Wimpy bar only lasted a few months. The messing around was getting worse and the manager told me to leave his premises and pick up my wages that weekend. From there I signed on the dole, and lived on that with great difficulty and guilt.

Every night I was out on the lash, drinking, in other words. I was getting fed up of always being on the receiving end of a tongue lashing from my mother – 'Where were you Liz, why didn't you come home last night? You're grounded, no more going out this week.' I had to shimmy down the drain pipe to meet my mates. My legs would be bruised and cut. To make it worse, I could never climb back up the damn drain pipe to my bedroom due to the Pony drinks making my two legs hollow. This meant I had to eat humble pie and knock on the front door, or throw pebbles at her window to try and wake her up, depending on how late at night it was. Mam was very worried about me, and would tell everyone that would listen what a devil I was for making her worry and lose her sleep.

I had it all planned, my great escape. First I asked Aunt Biddy – that was a no go, because her son was staying with them. She told me to stay where I was until I had a deposit on the rent for a nice place to live. Biddy didn't understand my predicament, though. I was to stay in and not go out every night? Blow that! I thought. I'm young and ready to enjoy my life going out and having a laugh with my friends. The Evening Advertiser advertised every week rooms to rent, some of which were rough and shoddy-looking places, very near public houses. A room was advertised one Tuesday afternoon. I rang the landlord, an Italian man called Giuseppe. He required two weeks' rent in advance. Once he got that, I could move in straight away.

Aunt Biddy helped me out with finance, and the room was mine: I had my first rent book. It was a bit dingy. I disliked it terribly. It wasn't like my home – no Mammy to wait on me, hand, foot and finger. This was the real world, and hey, I did not like what I found. However, I stayed there for over seven long weeks, being a stubborn little madam. Although it was only forty-nine days, to me it seemed forever; but I wasn't going home too soon.

I did miss Ma and three-year-old Anna, big time. But no way would I go home with my tail between my legs, to let Mammy know I had made a huge mistake. She even begged me to come back home, promising to buy me a radio-tape recorder for myself. I could see Frank's face making a frowned look, and that was it: I was going home for some TLC, and to torment the quare fella himself on the sly!

By God, it was great to be home that night in my nice warm cosy bed, with the crisp clean sheets and pillow cases. Mam had gotten Frank to paint my bedroom for me, and she bought new flowered linoleum to match the walls and curtains. God bless my dear mother. All the torture I put her through and she still spoiled me rotten. Unconditional love she showered on me. At times I felt bad for tormenting people. I really didn't know how or why I could do this to the ones I loved and adored, my dear family: Mam, Frank, young Anna and the other relatives in Swindon.

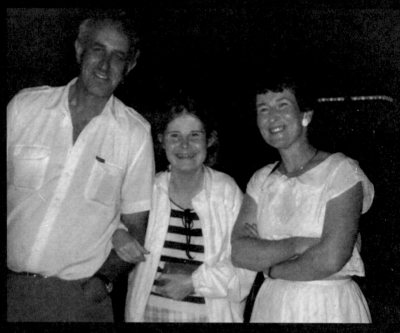

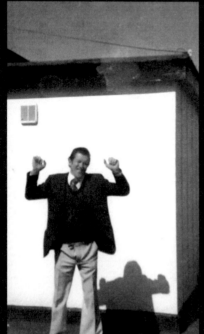

Above:
My Uncle Davy, Aunt Patty and myself
after the second transplant. I nearly died
and spent 12 weeks in hospital, including
a week in intensive care. I had a cardiac
arrest.

Left:
Nedser the Gambler.

Facing page, from top:
A happy memory: Me and Mam outside
The Ship in Swanage, Sept 1981.

Aunty Patty and me.

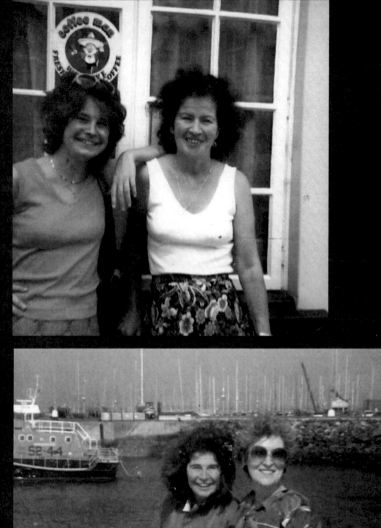
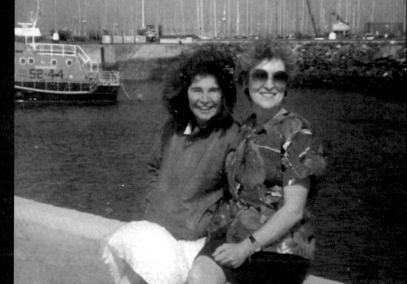

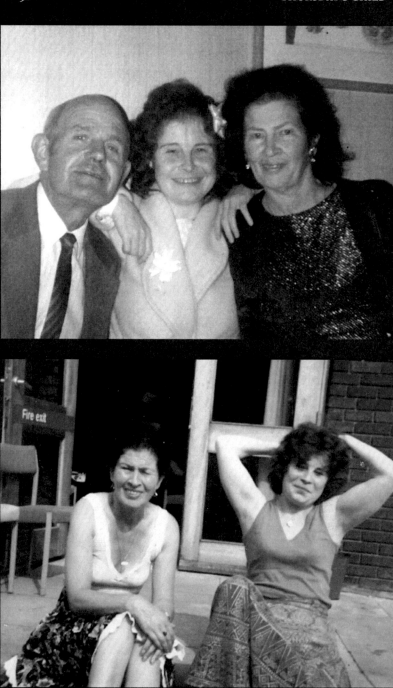

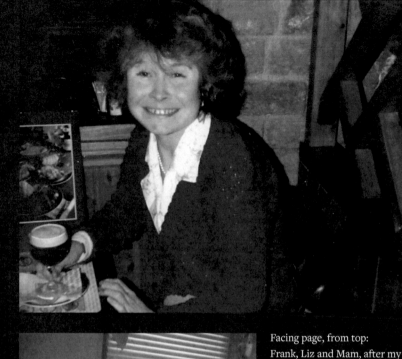

Facing page, from top:
Frank, Liz and Mam, after my successful third transplant.

After dialysis in my twenties.

This page, from top:
My birthday in The Running Horse, 1987.

Lizzybits on dialysis.

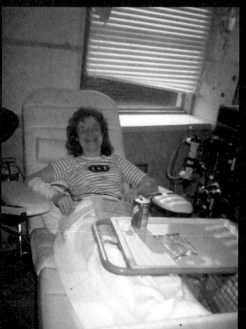

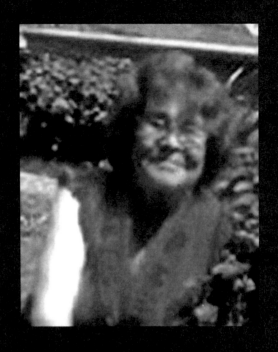

Part Four

All my Blessings:
Life with Chronic Renal Failure

The months went on and my kidneys were really hurting and stinging me. I woke one morning. Holy God, I thought I had gone blind. My sight was blurred and my head was in severe pain. The local GP sent me to the hospital for a check-up; they admitted me. From there I was sent to Oxford Kidney Hospital. They found I was near to complete renal failure. Soon my body would need a kidney dialysis machine. I was in stage two; when I reached four that would be it! The high blood pressure tablets worked and my eyesight came good again. It was great to be able to see out of my two eyes again. Thank you, God.

Now I was to go to the clinic in Oxford once every few months, but once I was discharged, I never bothered again. Who did they think they were, telling Elizabeth how to run her life? 'Blow me down with a feather duster! I have a life to live.' Or so I thought, but over the next year or so I got very ill. I was supposed to stick to a low sodium, potassium, phosphorus diet, as well as a fluid restriction. But if I saw it, I ate or drank it – that was my new diet! As for taking my much needed tablets, yeah right, forget that. Eventually my body was shutting down on me. Some days I was unable to leave my bed, or walk down the stairs. Mam would call me for my bacon rasher sandwich. It was very unlike me not to be up and dressed. Usually, to get me up, all Ma needed to do was fry a rasher on the pan. She knew that would always rouse me from my bed.

It went back to the time of my childhood. Grandad would be up cleaning the Stanley range on a Saturday or Sunday morning; he took great pride in his job. When he was finished, he cleaned the pan and found the dripping to fry the breakfast. The minute Galtee rashers started sizzling on that pan, it was like the exodus: we all started making our way down the stairs for the full Irish. The kettle would be on for our tea, the whistle just starting to whirr; the breakfast all plated up ready to serve, the bread cut and buttered all ready to be devoured by the hungry family. Grandad was great. Mind you, he would want our praise for jobs well done: 'The range looks great, Grandad.' 'The food tasted lovely.' 'Thank you very much' was all he needed to make him happy. Grandad was worth his weight in gold, no matter what state he was in after his heavy drinks on a Friday night.

Mam was getting very worried. I was unable to stay awake through the day. I was losing my appetite and couldn't keep any food or drink down. Now I know my system was well messed up with my anorexia nervosa, but this was genuinely serious. My two wonderful kidneys were at the end of their day: end-stage chronic renal failure. The words of my doctor in Ireland came back to haunt my Ma and me. In the early 1960s, when I was very young, he told her that I would need a kidney machine to keep me alive. In those days, people had never heard of these life-saving machines. If a patient's kidneys stopped working, they died and that was it. There was no life-saving kidney machine keeping their bodies going by cleaning their blood of toxic waste.

The way that I was feeling now was terrible. I couldn't pee very well. The pain in my kidneys and the stinging in my bladder and uterus when I passed water was excruciating. The tears would stream down my pale face. Mammy decided one day to bring me out for a Sunday spin. Frank drove us to Park South, to the Cock Robin public house in Cavendish Square. A local Irish group always played there for a few hours at lunchtime. I was sitting there, yet I was in another world entirely. I must have dozed off, because next minute my head hit down on the table. The glasses went crashing on the floor. The landlord came rushing over to our table and spoke quietly to Mammy. He told her nicely to take me home, that I was drunk or on drugs. I was in a stupor alright, not from drink but from toxins on my brain.

That was it for Mam. She decided she was getting me the help I desperately needed. She called our own doctor, but he refused point blank to come near me. This was because of my obnoxious and rude behaviour over the last few years. He once told me I would be dead before my nineteenth birthday, that no doctor would bother to treat me for my rudeness and argumentativeness. It was now four months past my nineteenth birthday, and I was extremely ill and very near death. Maybe the doctor's prediction would be right after all.

At that moment, all I wanted was to lie down somewhere away from everyone and quietly die. With that, Mammy called 999 to get me an ambulance. I was rushed into hospital in Swindon, and from there I was transferred immediately, blue light flashing, all the way to the Churchill Hospital for the Renal Nephrology doctors to get me on the desperately needed treatment.

Chronic End Stage Kidney Failure

I was admitted to the Renal Unit in the Churchill Hospital, Headington, Oxford. I cannot remember much. Everything was a complete blank until a loud buzzing noise woke me up after a good sleep. There was a dreadful pain in my head. Standing to the right beside my bed was a big noisy machine draped in tubes. These plastic tubes had blood inside them.

'Well now, I think it's my blood,' I thought, 'because this tube is new and it's in my neck. Aw God, where's my mother? This is too much for me to cope with on my own. What in God's name is happening to me?'

'Nurse help me please, get me off this contraption this minute. Where's my mother, Nurse? Please.'

'Calm down now, Elizabeth,' she told me.

'My name is Lizzy,' I told her.

'That's my name too', she said, trying to cajole me along. Then she explained that the tube access I had in my neck was now my only lifeline. Without this treatment I was going to die. The vascular access was making my life-saving haemodialysis possible. Haemodialysis is a life-saving treatment for kidney disease and kidney failure that uses a mechanical machine to send the blood through a filter, called a dialyser, outside the body.

I was given a fistula in my wrist. This is a surgically created vein used to remove and return blood during haemodialysis. The blood goes through an arterial needle, a few ounces at a time. The blood then travels through a tube that takes it to the dialyser. Inside this dialyser, the blood flows through very fine thin fibres; these filter out toxic wastes and any extra fluid. The machine then returns my clean filtered blood to my body through a different tube. The vascular access allows large amounts of my blood to flow continuously during the five hour haemodialysis session. Roughly a pint of blood flows through my machine every minute.

By rights, my vascular access should have been put in place a good few weeks or even months before I was due to go on my machine. My veins were never good for getting any blood. Even a normal blood test was a trial. The fistula failed within two days, so the consultant brought me back to theatre and inserted another one on the other wrist. Arrrrrrrrr, that was a joke too. The pain in my wrists! My veins were horrors for me.

June 16, 1979. That's when I started on my long journey of kidney failure. Haemodialysis for five hours at a time every Monday, Wednesday, and Friday afternoon for ten long years. Not long after starting on dialysis, the doctor asked me if I would like to do my treatment at home in Swindon. This would save me travelling by ambulance to my treatment thirty-six or so miles away. They could set it up in my bedroom, or they could erect a Portacabin hut in my mother's back garden, providing Swindon Borough Council gave the hospital the go ahead. My mother was going to be my carer and she would be paid to be my care assistant.

Everything got the go ahead, and Mam said yes to the doctors, so our training began six months later in my newly erected Portacabin. It was really wonderful for me having this mini life-saving hospital in our garden. My kidney machine was bought and paid for by the Six

Counties Renal Association and the Patient's Trust in the Churchill Renal Unit. I will be forever grateful to all the sponsors.

One morning, my dear mother put me on the machine. She was a bit tired and stressed, and she was rushing because I needed to come off a bit early that particular morning. As she was taking the arterial tube out, she went to pick up the clamp that usually lay side by side with the scissors, in the methylated spirits mixture used to sterilise the instruments needed for tube connection and disconnection. Next minute, we both let out a high-pitched roar. My arterial line was pumping blood. It was going everywhere – up the wall, on the bed, up to the ceiling, over our clothes. Mammy had only picked up the scissors and cut through my arterial line thinking she had clamped it! I felt myself going dizzy with shock and loss of blood. We managed to prevent me bleeding to death, by just about managing to get the plastic clamp and give it a good squeeze shut to stop the blood, and by stopping the haemodialysis pump.

Getting the much needed blood back to my body was trickier. Hospital help was needed. Thank God for British Telecom. Of course, Mam was crying her eyes out, nearly hysterical. I gave her an Anxicalm which I kept hidden for stressful times. This was to help her cope while she was getting step by step coaching on the phone to get me off the machine manually before the blood all clotted. Thank God, she made a great job of it. We were both complete and utter nervous wrecks. I was praying under my breath Mam would be okay – she was a born worrier. The few prayers calmed me down.

Anyway, back it was to travelling to Oxford three days a week, for years to come. How true it is about Thursday's Child. I had far to go.

Peritoneal Dialysis

A few years later, I tried the peritoneal dialysis. This was a bag system attached to a permacatheter in my peritoneal. This was placed in my lower tummy and I did these bag changes every four hours without fail, with eight hours rest overnight. My tummy was huge and really swelled up with the two litres of fluid I had to carry around all day, and it was very hard to walk any distance at all. But when things were all going well, I loved this peritoneal dialysis treatment. It was more like normal reality than going on a dialysis machine five hours at a time, three days per week. 'PD', as it was nicknamed, seemed nice and relaxed to me.

I could head off on holidays without any worry about finding a dialysis unit that could fit me in as a holiday patient. I could choose the holiday destination, ring the Six Counties Renal Association and they fixed everything up. The boxes were delivered to where I was headed, no problem at all. How cool was that for a renal patient on life-saving treatment?

Lots of fun was had. Milford-on-Sea caravan park near Bournemouth. Weekends in Bath on Avon and Harlow in Essex. My mother took me to Jersey with her for a week's holiday. I even travelled to my family in Dublin City for a few weeks! It was ace to be able to go off gallivanting when and where I liked, within reason of course. We would just load up the car boot with the peritoneal bags, and all that was needed was to do my four daily changes, plus two hot water bottles and large towels to warm the bags in case they were too cold and gave me the shivers. Cold bags could cause tummy cramp, or even the squirts in the night. I would boil a kettle, fill up the hot water bottles with boiling water, and wrap them in the towels to heat my CAPD bags.

Over the years I got a few doses of peritonitis – a terrible bad poison that attacks the walls of the tummy. I needed strychnine or rat poison to treat this. After my second kidney transplant I had the last dose; it took seven weeks to cure it. I would be roaring with the pain when the Pethedine injection wore off, and the nurses had to run to get me injected again, so I wouldn't upset the other patients on the ward. I honestly could not help the antics, so I needed to go back on the kidney dialysis machine again! This carried on year after year. I was now twenty-seven years old and, with my hardships in life, very hateful of everything. Without dialysis I was a goner. Depression set in; feeling sorry for myself. My dear mother was driven up the wall with the carry on out of me.

Bashful Barney
Barney the bashful Irish man was shy until he had a pint or two of Carling Black Label. This was sure to loosen his tongue and get his larynx into a singing tone. Then nothing pleased him more than a bit of banter and a

good old singsong like years before, when he was a youngster singing at hooleys in the kitchen in the mid-1940s in Ireland. When people egged him on with applause and asked him to sing another song, he loved it and got louder and put in more facial expressions. He clearly loved telling me these stories, the first night we met. In olden days people were more family orientated. Neighbours would all congregate in each other's humble abodes for nights of music and dance, to make merry and enjoy their own banter, chats, poetry and recitations, as if they hadn't heard the same things week after week for many moons. The applause would be deafening just the same, making the performer feel overjoyed. Once started it was a job to whist someone up, or let anyone else get a go at entertaining the audience. Most household members played musical instruments, and very well too, even if it was only a mouth organ.

Money for booze was not on the priority list in those times. An odd time someone might sneak in a bottle of Poteen. This was banned in Ireland due to it being a lethal brew. It's made from grain, beet, molasses, sugar, whey and good old Irish potatoes. The kilns were usually hidden well out of sight, where guards would not think of going to look – in the wood or in barns covered in straw bales, way back out of view.

It started with a kiss, and that after my kissing too many old bull frogs and toads. I wasn't looking for any long lasting relationship, that's for sure. I was young and looking for fun, laughter and whatever else came along the way, so I didn't think too much about this new man. There was a big Irish dance on in the sports centre in Stratton Street Market, in honour of blessed Saint Patrick. Frank was now working in Wales on a building site, and struck up a friendship with this Barney fellah. Frank decided to bring him up to meet his family in Swindon. With the Irish dance on, we knew it was a great excuse for them to have a good night out with free bed and breakfast thrown in. The dance was a great event, Barney informed me. He talked about the crowds from Reading, Bristol and other areas who often travelled to these Irish dances by hired coaches. We chatted about the singer Philomena Begley, how good she was. She was playing at the dance that evening.

For some reason I didn't fancy going, because Eddie, the guy I was after, was meant to be meeting me in the usual place. It was the usual evening out for me, sitting in my pub. I called it mine because I spent most of my life there. I was like the queen of the silver dollar. A wine glass was my sceptre, the bar stool was my throne. To be sitting there watching over my kingdom was a thrill, or so I thought in my sad hammered mind.

The men missed their train back to Wales, or so they told us. They were at home when I got in late from my rendezvous with romance. Mam waited for me to get home, then headed off to her bed. Frank had the tapes blasting out. Margo O'Donnell was singing 'Donegal Shore' at the top of her voice. I went to turn her down, in case the noise woke my little sister Anna Marie. Well, Frank grabbed the tape recorder out of my hand. I let fly at him, and threw a few curses for good measure. He went off to bed in disgust.

Barney looked gobsmacked, but we got chatting about our lives and the people in it. He told me about his early years. He was christened Daniel, but an old man of the road, who would call to buy fish from his grandparents every time he was visiting the coastal village, for some reason always called young Daniel by the name Barney. To this day, the nickname stuck with him. His grandparents brought the young boy up. Barney painted a great picture of his early childhood days: the shenanigans with the school lads in the village of Bonmahon, the fun and games with his cousin John Dwan, and the fooling around they would get up to. Coming from a fishing community, all the large family of Dwans were into the fishing in some way. The uncles went out in their boats, catching the mackerel in the summer months, and pollock or other fish at other times. They would sell the fish at the door of their home. These old ways are well gone. Barney told me the history of the miners that mined for copper underneath the village and way out to sea. Bonmahon sounded a lovely place to live.

Eventually, after hours of chatting about everything, we were worn out, but a swift kiss was given before I headed off to my bed, happy and tired after the long gossip half the night. God, my throat was sore from all the fags we smoked. Barney chain smoked, as did I myself. I threw him a few blankets to keep him warm, and a pillow to rest his weary head. I even put the gas fire on for him to keep him warm! God if Mam had caught me doing that, wasting gas on a stranger, she would have had my guts for garters.

The two men were heading home early to try and make a half shift on the building site. I thought no more about Barney or his elaborate stories of his village life by the sea.

Rollercoaster Life

I was travelling three days a week for my treatment now. Sometimes if I got a bad clot in my tube I would need to go in for de-clotting. First I had it in my leg, then my neck, now my arm, which clotted more, don't ask me why. I would be brought into the haemodialysis unit by ambulance car transport. Alan, my favourite dialysis technician, would hot-rod my dialysis tube: big long wires were put up to the top of my arm, and a balloon would be blown up to pull down the veins. Did it hurt? God yes, it pained like hell! I would try not to cry my eyes out, much as I wanted to. I didn't want the nice looking technicians to think I was a wuss. They would always say how brave and courageous I was. This always cheered me up – I loved praise of any kind, because I felt I never got it when it was needed, growing up. If they couldn't unblock my arm they had to keep me in hospital on the dialysis ward.

One weekend, out of the blue, Barney arrived up to the Churchill Hospital on the Saturday afternoon. To say I was shocked was an understatement. Not many of those frogs or toads bothered coming to visit me when I was in hospital all those years. It made me feel extra special that someone other than my family was coming all the way from Wales to visit me. We went to Headington, the nearby town. There was a big match on between Oxford and some other town, and the riot police were out in force in case mayhem broke out. We went into a foreign restaurant and had a Moroccan meal. We ate Moussaka. I didn't like it, but I pretended I did because Barney had bought it for me. Neither of us had tasted this food before, and I think we were bluffing, eating every bit. Gosh, did I feel bloated and nauseous! The hospital only gave me an hour and a half out, but we managed to have a couple of drinks in the Britannia, and get away before the match ended in case we got held up in any fracas. Going back I felt happy and merry.

That week seemed to pass by quickly enough; they allowed me home the following Friday afternoon, and up comes my bashful prince Barney for the weekend! After that, when we weren't together, we phoned each other regularly, without fail.

Months passed. We had our fair share of drinking at weekend parties in Rodbourne Road, with my mother and Frank. The Irish tapes would be blasting out 'Shannongolden' and Margo would be singing 'Donegal Shore' and Brendan Shine would be singing out 'Hey Louise', or young Daniel O'Donnell was away with 'The Old Rugged Cross'. That was my mother's favourite song. She would shed the odd tear, bless her, as we supped, listened and sang along to them all.

Then the rows started between Mam and me. She was a periodic binge drinker. The binges would go on for weeks at a time. Life was like a rollercoaster – up and down, fun and games, weekends away and mad drinking sessions and of course the odd few rows for good measure! The rows were always from drink...

Barney was still living down in Wales. I was ready to move away, so off I went down to Gwent. It was a lovely place, but soon I was homesick. After getting a bout of peritonitis in my tummy from the dialysis, it was a case of having to go home whether I wanted to or not. I was too far away from Oxford and the Renal Unit. After a while I got my own flat near west Swindon, where I stayed for years. Drink played havoc with me at times. I always seemed to love abusing my body with booze, cigarettes and the odd pain reliever for good measure.

Barney came up from Wales one weekend. He went over to my friend's house across the road; they were having a party. I didn't go with him. Back he comes with a bitch! This dog belonged to a friend of a friend of ours. They didn't want her anymore, which I thought was awful. Barney carried the dog over the road in his arms for me. I was so chuffed! I was sure this dog would run home to her old house but no, she never did. Gemma was her name.

Oh my God, I loved this wonderful crossed Collie Springer. She was about seven years old when she came to my flat to live. We became best buddies. We were inseparable. My loyal dog walked miles on end with me talking to her, telling her all my woes. She would know how to console me when we got home: she would saunter over to me, staring at me with her soppy eyes and resting her loving chin on my knees, trying to tell me she was there for me. Gemma helped me through ten years of counselling for my binges. You see, whenever I got stressed I needed booze, full stop, and nothing would stop me getting it, even if I spent the electric money.

I had one good friend, let's call this woman 'Suckee put the kettle on'. She lived across the road from my flat in Moredon. We had some laughs and high jinx – 'One was bad, the other worse'. We could drink the bar dry if we weren't watched. We loved cooking and I often spent hours pouring over her cookery books. We were best pals.

Suckee was with me in 1987 when the call came for my second kidney transplant. She took the call as I was out. When I came home, Suckee had the hospital bag packed for me. I was very nervous and anxious, yet excited. Next thing the ambulance medicar arrived to escort me up to the transplant unit. My tummy was doing cartwheels. I passed all the tests for having the kidney. There were two: a guy I know got the other kidney. I did an exchange on my peritoneal dialysis. After I signed the form to let them go ahead with the transplant, they gave me my pre-med before going to theatre: I felt lovely and woozy, like I was merry.

It was all a haze to me: I remember doctors running with the trolley and then nothing. I thought I was dead. A beautiful white light was in front of me; it felt like I was flying without wings. I felt at peace, without cares or worries. I kept drifting to this white light. I honestly didn't want to come back to my body – that's where my stresses and strains and suffering and pain belonged. Up here, I was in heaven.

I had had three major operations in three days. A ventilator was breathing for me, and now they were turning my ventilator off, so it was fingers crossed for my survival. The next fourteen hours were critical. There was now no more white mist. That made me sad. I loved the feeling of oblivion I felt in this beautiful place. When the pain relief wore off, the pain in my stomach was excruciating. I would be roaring in agony. The doctor told me I had peritonitis in my tummy. The infection was in my bag system. I wanted to die; the pain was too much for me to bear. It was seven weeks before they could get a proper antibiotic – Streptomycin. This started working almost straight away, thank goodness. My tummy was all scarred inside, so a new access line was put in my neck, called a permacath.

I didn't like being back on my haemo machine. I was in hospital for 12 weeks altogether. My aunt and uncle came over from Ireland to visit me. They got a mighty shock at the sight of me. I looked like death warmed up, they told Mam. After getting out of hospital I went home to recuperate. I was too weak and poorly to get around. Finally Gemma and I went back to live in the flat in Moredon. Suckee helped and kept me company for a while. I was going up and down to Oxford for over three years afterwards.

'I have had enough!' I told them. 'To hell with it. I cannot do this any more, I have had enough of this renal life.'

Depression had set in big time. I suffered very badly. I often felt going to sleep that never waking up would be bliss. It scared me to get these awful thoughts. Not Barney, my family or even Gemma could help me. So I told Dr Oliver I had had enough. There was an emergency meeting called – a big powwow of transplant and renal doctors. The talk about Liz McCue went on for ages before finally it was decided I was to be given the benefit of the doubt. Another transplant might make me better and maybe stop my bingeing on drink. The doctor called me into his office.

'We need to give you this pager. You're now on call twenty-four hours. You must continue on dialysis until a kidney arrives. The pager could go at any time of the day or night, Liz. Stick with us now and keep yourself well, just in case a kidney comes.'

I had hope at last.

Kidney Transplant

Two weeks later the pager beeped. Holy Mary Mother of God my heart did somersaults inside my ribcage. Aw, the excitement I felt! Euphoria! Everything worked out to perfection: Yes, the kidney was a great match for me. I had the op.

The very next day I was up and about! It felt like I had been re-born again in a healthy body. For once there was no severe depression. Okay I was a little bit sore – who wouldn't be after a big four hour op in theatre? It felt wonderful to be able to have a proper piss, instead of a dribble now and again. It felt like I was in heaven. No more horrid life-saving kidney dialysis machine keeping me alive. Oh no, now I had my own beautiful grafted kidney.

How blessed I felt. This was better than all the riches in the world. Having good health was blissful. When I thought of all the stress kidney failure caused me, it made me even more grateful to the kidney donor that left me the healthy hard-working kidney.

To people reading this chapter, my gratitude goes to all kidney donors who donate their organs to give another person the wonderful Gift of Life. Unless your life depended on a transplant, then you could never imagine the gratitude or the divine love that is felt for the donor that helps save the life of a kidney patient. To me, getting that successful kidney felt like I had won a million on the Lotto. Everything is possible having good health. Yes, I believe it's true that our health is our wealth!

After having the transplant, I started to travel. I toured around England, Wales and parts of Ireland. Barney had his own twenty-one foot boat called a punt. He had it in the local dock near Boatstrand, which in Irish is Dunabrattin. In the summertime he would go fishing for mackerel and in the winter he would head back to England to carry on the building work. He was a great worker and could turn his hand to anything. He always had work in England or Wales. Life was never boring and it was fun to be able to head off on excursions whenever he could come up to see me. Everything was going great!

Family Turmoil

In 1995 my sister Anna was to turn twenty-one. With the fourteen year difference between us, this gave me my thirty-fifth birthday on the same day. We were having a surprise party for my sister. My mother and I were kept busy. A friend of the family, a lovely guy by the name of Albert, was helping us put on the party, as we could never afford a huge big buffet and a disco. Thanks Albert for bringing us together. This was very kind and thoughtful of you. The party went with a bang, but Mam was looking a bit off colour – a bit grey, and she felt sick. She headed home early. Often Louie suffered with irritable bowel and had bad bouts now and then. Maybe she had just eaten something to turn her tummy.

We were going to a funeral the next morning, for a dear old family friend's wife, RIP. Usually we would go for a cup of tea, and a bite to eat afterwards. Mammy was in desperate agony, with her neck pain and her tummy. This neck pain had been going on constantly. Deep heat was never far from her – the times I rubbed it on for her, God bless her heart. We caught the bus home, and I left her off at her stop and carried on home. That night the phone rang around eleven. It was Mammy ringing to say goodnight, letting me know the pain was a bit easier. I was glad to hear it, and I headed off to my bed.

The next morning around half past nine, the phone woke me with a start.

'Liz come down quick I need you now urgently. I will explain when you come down to me. Please come quickly.'

God bless her, she was in a state by the time I arrived to the house. Thank God the door was easy to open. Mam had fallen out of bed. Her legs wouldn't hold her up. She could not get up to walk so she shimmed down the stairs on her rump. When she got to the phone, she could pull herself up by the table leg as it was sturdy. She couldn't remember my number – her mind was all fuzzy and hazy – so she rang my number by pressing the redial button.

I called 999 at half past eleven. When the ambulance arrived much later, Mammy wouldn't get in; she refused point blank. Then at two I rang the doctor to explain the situation. The minutes seemed like hours and my mother was deathly pale. The pain in her neck was excruciating. I rubbed loads of deep heat into her neck and shoulders. At last, the doctor came after surgery at half past six, and persuaded her to go in for a check up. The nurse in charge rang me and told me to get myself to the hospital quickly. Ten minutes after being assessed by an A & E doctor, our dear mother had fallen into a coma!

Some days later, God took our mother to heaven. She had been on a life support machine since admission. An aneurysm caused our mother to have two mini strokes and a full stroke. If Louie had come through the coma, her mind and body would not have functioned and a wheelchair would have been needed 24/7. Oh God, how I cried. Buckets.

You see, in a way, I knew my mother was going to die. The family all refused to believe this, but I knew, because I had dreamt it the morning before the terrible accident. In my life-like dream, the coffin was going deep into the soil. It was me that lay in this coffin, not my mother. My mother and sister were miles away. I was losing them both. They looked down at me, and then they turned and just walked away. I tried calling them from the grave, but no-one heard my cries. All this really happened, only it was our mother in the coffin going deep underground. She couldn't hear Anna or me calling her.

Part of my soul died after the burial of our dear mother Louise Mary Smith, RIP. The funeral was held up for weeks because of terrible weather. Torrential rain filled graves as quickly as they were dug. This was heart breaking. To have lost my mother was severe enough. Having to wait twenty-eight days to bury her was too much for us to bear. God, life can be very tough. To think that a couple of months earlier, we were excitedly planning the birthday bash for Anna's twenty-first. As I stood there like a lost soul, family and dear friends throwing flowers on top of her beautiful coffin, this heartbreak took me hard.

Anna had a bit of a meltdown. Not surprising, considering all the care my mother had given her daughter Anna and her grandchild Scotty, who was an adorable little boy, but a right handful at the best of times. His dear Nana Louie could humour the little chap no problem at all, and adored the ground Scotty walked on, as we all did; he was a darling boy. After our mother Louie died, young Scotty went to stay with his loving grandparents. But that's another story.

My sweet sister suffered constantly with manic depression and severe panic attacks. At times she could just about cope with herself alone, never mind trying to look after her little two-year-old child. We had a slight dispute about the child after our Mam died, and other things. So really the nightmare I had did come true: I lost them both – my mother to death and my sister for a short while to bipolar disorder. That dream was a warning to me. I get those dreams when things go wrong in my family life. Thank God, after a certain period of time, our bond was mended. Now hell or high water will never break my sister and I up ever again. I would die for her as if she was my own child. That's how much I love my darling sister Anna. A couple of years after Mam died, Anna met her other half. They decided to have a baby. First came a lovely baby boy and later a little girl. I was so happy for them.

The Return to Ireland

A few years later, it was decided Barney and I would return to Ireland for the summer. We bought this nifty looking car, a nice little run around, from a garage near Blunsdon. They certainly had a great laugh at our expense, that's for sure. Oh the car looked the part alright, but half way down to Wales a bearing went in the front wheel. Oh my God! We had Gemma the dog, Teasy Weasy the stray cat, our colour television, and pots and pans to use in the caravan in sunny Tramore, County Waterford. We got the car as far as the motorway services in Pont Abraham, sat down and decided on our next move over a couple of cups of tea. We rang a few places that fixed motorcars. The prices we were given to get the car towed to a local garage, well let's say it was extremely overpriced! But it had to be fixed, and there was a lot more wrong than just a bearing, that's for sure. We were stranded.

We stayed in our car overnight. That saved us a hotel or bed and breakfast stay. We had loads of duvets and blankets to keep us warm. The animals were well fed and well watered. The cat played silly devils hiding under cars on me – I was nearly crying until finally out came Teasy Weasy, the brazen little pussykins, nice as you like – 'meaow meaow' – looking for her next plate of grub.

We ordered a taxi to take us to the nearest pub, which served mouth-watering food that was warming and nourishing. We chatted about what to do next. Certainly, getting to Ireland was a big No! We were heading home along the M4 Motorway like two old dogs that lost their tails. We were truly raging not to be able to go on our excursion to the Emerald Isle.

So, it was back to the drawing board for our second attempt at the plan. On the Irish bank holiday May 1, it was all stations go. We set sail with the menagerie, television, radio, pots, pans and anything else we could put in the new car for comfort.

The months drifted by. I never did go home to England. I stayed in the sunny southeast. First in an eight-berth caravan in Tramore for a couple of months in the early season. I loved every minute of this wonderful time. It reminded me of my summer holidays spent with my dear mother Louie in County Galway...

The woman my mother worked for was a music teacher. She taught the piano. This woman's husband was a medical professor. A couple of years running, they brought my mother and me with their children down to their big holiday house beside the sea in Salthill, just outside Galway City. It was heavenly for me having playmates as a child. My mother's responsibility was to care for the children and take them out in the day time. The professor and his wife were working all week in Dublin, and returning to the holiday home for their weekends. I had a lovely few holidays there as a child.

So, beautiful sunny Tramore was perfect for me with its sandy beach, the kayaking and surfers, walkers and swimmers out enjoying the bright summer nights.

After that we moved to Barney's relation's flat that they rented out. It was really great having a kidney transplant. To say it was 'bliss to piss' might sound crude, but until one cannot wee, one will not understand my pun. Not needing some form of treatment to keep me alive was really awesome to me. For over thirteen long happy years I gave great gratitude for the person that died and gave me this extra precious gift of life. I had been ready to give up my long struggle, and all the stresses and strains of chronic end-stage renal failure. Thank God for organ donation. To the people who donate their organs or even leave parts or all their bodies to medical science, sincere gratitude is sent to all, and their thoughtful grieving families. It cannot be very easy for them to make that decision.

Eventually, however, my body started to swell up. My face, legs, ankles, throat, you name it. I felt puffed all over. I felt tired, itchy, fatigued, contrary – just really miserable. I couldn't walk very far from the flat. To eat or drink became unappetising and often I was sick. Everyone noticed how unwell I looked. My hospital visits were two-monthly, and after the last clinic I was to come every two weeks. Eventually I was called in to the clinic, after a blood test showed that my creatinine, urea and potassium had shot up rapidly. Urgent treatment was needed.

Dublin sent for me to attend the ward the next day. I was gutted. A very sad day, going back on the life-saving haemodialysis machine yet again. There were good times, great times, awful times and stressed-out times.

Finding my Angels

I visited Lourdes in 2010, the start of my spiritual journey with the angels. From then on, good things started happening to me. I never was much into spiritual stuff through my booze-fuelled years. I had no time for mumbo jumbo, as I put it in those times. After the Lourdes pilgrimage, I started attending Mass. This brought calm into my mind, thankfully. I met a beautiful woman from Bonmahon, an English lady. Her husband knew my other half, Barney. They were fishermen through the years. I often called to her house for tea and spiritual chats about our angels. We loved these meet-ups and I borrowed lots of Angel books from Audrey O'Reilly. The hours on my haemodialysis machine melted away and a peace filled my soul. Positivity took over and negativity flew out through my crown chakra. Life was good. I started looking out for other people. I was on Facebook for years and I decided to set up my own angel page. It was called Lizzybits Angel Passenger Pals. I picked out all my positive pals from my timeline page. These friends could add a few friends of their own. I started with one friend, now there are 245! The only rules are: no swearing, no misery, no abusing other members. Random acts of kindness and plenty of prayers are said for all members. These can be done without using the person's name. We can also send distant Integrated Energy Therapy – an angelic healing energy that is used on points in our body.

I joined an Angel group in Dungarvan, County Waterford, run by a local person. This group is a psychic mediumship and healing group. There are a few girls that live near me and they pick me up in their car and take me the twelve miles to Dungarvan. We can all talk freely about our dreams and other experiences. It's great to have like-minded pals that are interested in Angels and healing with the hands. Sometimes all it needs is an ear to listen, a shoulder to cry on, a few kind words and a warm caring hug to heal other people. This group meets above a bar in Grattan Square. It's a very therapeutic room. We can practise on each other or we can do readings for each other. The organiser brought a new guy from Athboy, Edmond Carroll. He teaches the Integrated Energy Treatment. I have done the basic and the intermediate; next is the advanced, then the masters. If I do the final masters that means I can teach other students. I have two certificates to my name already!

I will be forever grateful to my darling friend Audrey for introducing me to my new spiritual path. My dear friend died in her fifties. She got the all-clear after her breast was removed; a couple of months later Audrey went to sleep with the Angels. To this day, every time I hear the song 'In the Arms of the Angels' I just know Audrey is connecting with my soul from Heaven. RIP my beautiful soul pal. I idolised the ground she walked on. I always felt at peace in Audrey's company. Their front room was a beautiful sanctuary for us both. We could talk for hours and never get tired or run out of chat.

As I say, there are lots of new doors opening for me in my new positive lifestyle. I no longer drink alcohol or smoke. I try to be kind to myself first and foremost. That way I can be of use to others by being kind, or just listening to their woes. That is all it needs sometimes. A caring friend, that is what I try to be to everyone that I meet and greet in my two lives – my dialysis life and my own outside life. Only for my life-saving kidney dialysis treatment three days a week for four hours at a time, I would also be in heaven long ago. Like my soul pal Audrey, I have had numerous meetings with the Divine since I was nineteen years old. However, the angels always take me back to mother Earth. I know I still have lots to do in this life – people to meet and help in some way or other.

Thanks to Sister Brenda our lovely nurse in charge, and also the Waterford Healing Arts Trust for giving me the amazing chance to write my autobiography. I have got great confidence since Philip Cullen came to our unit looking for patients to try their hand at art, poetry, etc. I was going to do photography. Next thing I know I'm half-way through my very own life story and himself is cracking the imaginary whip, 'keeping me on my toes' as he calls it. Oh yes, Mr Philip Cullen is a hard task master, and I appreciate him for it, because without his belief in my capability I would have fallen by the wayside after the first few chapters. God bless his heart, and also the wonderful art teacher Boyer Phelan from Stradbally. Over the years these lovely people have been a great help to me.

I have had a great healing coming to terms with some intolerable issues in my life. There were nights I couldn't sleep and other nights tossing and turning, not to mention writer's block! I put my heart and soul into this book. I shed tears of joy and sorrow. I hope that it might bring hope to someone out there. I want to let people know that life doesn't end when our kidneys fail. I am waiting on my fourth kidney transplant. Life for me is not a bowl of cherries, but I have great faith in my divine Angels and truly believe they are always with me as I struggle through the hard times. At times I can feel their soft feathery touch. The warm feeling on my left shoulder is them letting me know they are walking with me along my path on this beautiful spiritual journey.

When my time does come I can go with a clear conscience, knowing I did my best for others, even if I could have been kinder to my inner child at times. I look back and see that wonderful precious child that was afraid of letting her parents and grandparents down. Elizabeth would rather let herself down first. I remember all the nights I cried silently into the pillow, afraid to move in the bed in case a wallop from my father would catch me off guard, when a booze-fuelled temper came on him. It didn't happen often, thankfully, but I was afraid of my own shadow at times. Paul McKenna's CDs and books were a blessing in my older years and I can now stand up at our dialysis unit Thanksgiving Mass every year and give a reading from the pulpit. I have gained great confidence throughout the years.

I thank all of you truly, dear readers. I hope you enjoyed at least parts of my story and get hope, too, in some small way. I truly enjoyed writing it down, and if you like it, tell a friend. Whether you like or dislike my writing, please by all means tell me, on Facebook or Twitter. Love, light and angel blessings, from Lizzybits.